Gerda van Wezel-Meijler

Neonatal Cranial Ultrasonography

CW00869442

Gerda van Wezel-Meijler

Neonatal Cranial Ultrasonography

Guidelines for the Procedure and Atlas of Normal Ultrasound Anatomy

With 121 Figures and 1 Table

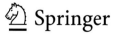 Springer

G. van Wezel-Meijler, MD, PhD, *pediatrician-neonatologist*
Department of Pediatrics, subdivision of Neonatology
Leiden University Medical Centre, J6-S
PO Box 9600
2300 RC Leiden
E-mail: G.van_Wezel-Meijler@lumc.nl

Illustrations by:
Lise Plamondon, *research nurse and medical illustrator*
Pavillon Desmarais # 2224
Department of Physiology (Medicine)
University of Montreal
C.P. 6128, Succ. C.V.
Montreal, Quebec
Canada H3C 3J7
E-mail: Lise.Plamondon@Umontreal.ca

Library of Congress Control Number: 2007921693
ISBN 978-3-540-69906-4 Springer Berlin Heidelberg New York

Springer-Verlag is a part of Springer Science+Business Media
springer.com
© Springer-Verlag Berlin Heidelberg 2007

Editor: Dr. Ute Heilmann, Heidelberg, Germany
Desk Editor: Meike Stoeck, Heidelberg, Germany
Typesetting and Production: LE-TEX Jelonek, Schmidt & Vöckler GbR, Leipzig, Germany
Cover Design: eStudio, Calamar, Spain

Printed on acid free paper   SPIN 12533428   21/3180/YL – 5 4 3 2 1

Contents

Acknowledgements

The author would like to thank:

- All the babies whose photographs and/or ultrasound scans are in this book
- The parents who gave permission to have pictures of their babies taken for educational purposes and publication
- Lise Plamondon, who, with endless patience, made the illustrations for this book and who was always willing to provide repetitive adjustments
- The staff and fellow neonatologists of the Department of Neonatology, Leiden University Medical Center
- The staff of the Department of Neuroradiology, Leiden University Medical Center
- Maurik Mietes and Esther van Wezel for their help with Reference Manager
- Frances Cowan and Linda de Vries

List of Abbreviations

CUS   Cranial Ultrasonography
DEHSI Diffuse Excessive High Signal Intensity
GA   Gestational Age
IPE   Intraparenchymal Echodensity
IVH   Intraventricular Haemorrhage
MHz   Megahertz
MR   Magnetic Resonance
MRI   Magnetic Resonance Imaging
NICU   Neonatal Intensive Care Unit
PCA   Post-Conceptional Age
PHVD Post-Haemorrhagic Ventricular Dilatation
P/IVH Peri-Intraventricular Haemorrhage
PLIC   Posterior Limb of Internal Capsule
PVL   Periventricular Leukomalacia
VI   Ventricular Index

Introduction

Cranial ultrasonography (CUS) was introduced into neonatology in the late 1970s and has become an essential diagnostic tool in modern neonatology. The non-invasive nature of ultrasonography makes it an ideal imaging technique in the neonate. In the neonate and young infant, the fontanels and many sutures of the skull are still open, and these can be used as acoustic windows to "look" into the brain. Transfontanellar CUS allows the use of high-frequency transducers, with high near-field resolution.

As a result of ongoing development in ultrasonography, image quality is high nowadays, provided optimal settings and techniques are applied. Therefore, CUS is a reliable tool for detecting congenital and acquired anomalies of the perinatal brain and the most frequently occurring patterns of brain injury in both preterm and full-term neonates.

This book is a practical guide to neonatal cranial ultrasonography.

The first part describes how to perform a standard, good-quality CUS procedure, using the anterior fontanel as an acoustic window. It continues with the application of supplemental acoustic windows (i.e. posterior fontanel, mastoid fontanels and the temporal windows). Recommendations are given on the timing of CUS examinations and on additional neuro-imaging (MRI).

The second part of the book deals with the normal anatomy of the neonatal brain as depicted by CUS. This is demonstrated using normal CUS images in different planes, obtained from different acoustic windows.

Although, in order to clarify some topics, examples of abnormal CUS images are shown, the focus of this book is on the normal ultrasound anatomy of the neonatal brain and on how to perform a good-quality

CUS examination. A systematic review of congenital and acquired anomalies of the neonatal brain as depicted by CUS is beyond the scope of this book. Recommendations are given for further reading on these subjects. Doppler and colour Doppler imaging are briefly mentioned; for more detailed information, the reader is referred to an earlier book on this subject *(Couture and Veyrac 2001)*.

The current book refers to some of the available literature on the subject of CUS, but it does not strive to give a complete overview of the literature. All ultrasound images were performed at the neonatal unit of the Leiden University Medical Center by the author of this book or one of her collegues, using an Aloka 5500 or Alpha 10 Ultrasound system.

The ultrasound images shown in this book are normal and age-appropriate unless stated otherwise.

The MRI examinations were performed at the department of neuroradiology of the Leiden University Medical Center, using Philips 1.5 or 3 Tesla MR systems.

Reference

1.   Couture A, Veyrac C. (2001) Transfontanellar Doppler imaging in neonates, 1st edn. Springer, Berlin

Further Reading

1.   Arthur R, Ramenghi LA (2001) Imaging the neonatal brain. In: Levene MI et al. (eds) Fetal and neonatal neurology and neurosurgery. Churchill Livingstone, London
2.   De Vries LS, Levene MI (2001) Cerebral ischemic lesions. In: Levene MI et al. (eds) Fetal and neonatal neurology and neurosurgery. Churchill Livingstone, London
3.   Govaert P, De Vries LS (1997) An atlas of neonatal brain sonography, 1st edn. MacKeith Press, Cambridge

4.   Levene MI (2001) The asphyxiated newborn infant. In: Levene MI et al. (eds) Fetal and neonatal neurology and neurosurgery. Churchill Livingstone, London

5.   Levene MI, De Vries LS (2001) Neonatal intracranial hemorrhage. In: Levene MI et al. (eds) Fetal and neonatal neurology and neurosurgery. Churchill Livingstone, London

6.   Levene MI et al. (1985) Ultrasound of the infant brain, 1st edn. Blackwell, Oxford

7.   Volpe JJ (2001a) Bacterial and fungal intracranial infections. In: Volpe JJ (ed) Neurology of the newborn. WB Saunders Company, Philadelphia

8.   Volpe JJ (2001b) Hypoxic-ischemic encephalopathy: clinical aspects. In: Volpe JJ (ed) Neurology of the newborn. WB Saunders, Philadelphia

9.   Volpe JJ (2001c) Intracranial hemorrhage: germinal matrix-intraventricular hemorrhage of the premature infant. In: Volpe JJ (ed) Neurology of the newborn. WB Saunders, Philadelphia

10.   Volpe JJ (2001d) Intracranial hemorrhage: subdural, primary subarachnoid, intracerebellar, intraventricular (term infant), and miscellaneous. In: Volpe JJ (ed) Neurology of the newborn. WB Saunders, Philadelphia

11.   Volpe JJ (2001e) Viral, protozoan, and related intracranial infections. In: Volpe JJ (ed) Neurology of the newborn. WB Saunders, Philadelphia

PART I

THE CRANIAL ULTRASOUND PROCEDURE

1 Cranial Ultrasonography: Advantages and Aims

1.1 Advantages of Cranial Ultrasonography

Major advantages of CUS are the following:

- It can be performed bedside, with little disturbance to the infant (*Fig. 1.1*); manipulation of the infant is hardly necessary.
- It can be initiated at a very early stage, even immediately after birth.

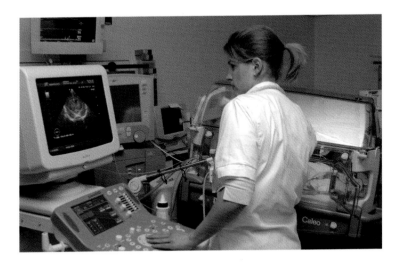

Fig. 1.1 Cranial ultrasound procedure performed in a premature infant in its incubator

- It is safe; (safety guidelines are provided by the British Medical Ultrasound Society www.bmus.org and the American Institute of Ultrasound in Medicine www.aium.com) *(British Medical Ultrasound Society 2006, American Institute of Ultrasound in Medicine 2006).*
- It can be repeated as often as necessary, and thereby enables visualisation of ongoing brain maturation and the evolution of brain lesions. In addition, it can be used to assess the timing of brain damage.
- It is a reliable tool for detection of most haemorrhagic, cystic, and ischaemic brain lesions as well as calcifications, cerebral infections, and major structural brain anomalies, both in preterm and full-term neonates.
- CUS is relatively inexpensive compared with other neuro-imaging techniques.
- For all these reasons it is an excellent tool for serial brain imaging during the neonatal period (and thereafter until closure of the fontanels).

1.2   Aims of Neonatal Cranial Ultrasonography

The aims of neonatal CUS are to assess
- Brain maturation
- The presence of structural brain abnormalities and/or brain injury
- The timing of cerebral injury
- The neurological prognosis of the infant

In seriously ill neonates and in neonates with serious cerebral abnormalities, either congenital or acquired, it plays a role in decisions on continuation or withdrawal of intensive treatment. In neonates surviving with cerebral injury, it may help to optimize treatment of the infant and support of the infant and his or her family, both during the neonatal period and thereafter.

Advantages of CUS	Aims of CUS

• Safe
 • Bedside- compatible
 • Reliable
 • Early imaging
 • Serial imaging:
   – Brain maturation
   – Evolution of lesions
 • Inexpensive
 • Suitable for screening
	• Exclude/demonstrate cerebral pathology
	 • Assess timing of injury
	 • Assess neurological prognosis
	 • Help make decisions on continuation of neonatal intensive care
	 • Optimise treatment and support

References

1. American Institute of Ultrasound in Medicine (2006) Standards for performance of the ultrasound examination of the infant brain. www.aium.com

2. British Medical Ultrasound Society (2006) Ultrasound in medicine. www.bmus.org

Further Reading

1. Ancel PY et al. (2006) Cerebral palsy among very preterm children in relation to gestational age and neonatal ultrasound abnormalities: the EPIPAGE cohort study. Pediatrics 117: 828–835

2. Arthur R, Ramenghi (2001) Imaging the neonatal brain. In: Levene MI et al. (eds) Fetal and neonatal neurology and neurosurgery. Churchill Livingstone, London

3. Bracci R et al. (2006) The timing of neonatal brain damage. Biol Neonate 90: 145–155

4. De Vries LS, Levene MI (2001) Cerebral ischemic lesions. In: Levene MI et al. (eds) Fetal and neonatal neurology and neurosurgery. Churchill Livingstone, London

5. De Vries LS, Groenendaal F (2002) Neuroimaging in the preterm infant. Ment Retard Dev Disabil Res Rev 8: 273–280

6.   De Vries LS et al. (1992) The spectrum of leukomalacia using cranial ultrasound. Behav Brain Res 49: 1–6

7.   De Vries LS et al. (2004a) The spectrum of cranial ultrasound and magnetic resonance imaging abnormalities in congenital cytomegalovirus infection. Neuropediatrics 35: 113–119

8.   De Vries LS et al. (2004b) Ultrasound abnormalities preceding cerebral palsy in high-risk preterm infants. J Pediatr 144: 815–820

9.   De Vries LS et al. (2006) The role of cranial ultrasound and magnetic resonance imaging in the diagnosis of infections of the central nervous system. Early Hum Dev 82: 819–825

10.   Govaert P, De Vries LS (1997) An atlas of neonatal brain sonography, 1st edn. MacKeith Press, Cambridge

11.   Leijser LM et al. (2004) Hyperechogenicity of the thalamus and basal ganglia in very preterm infants: radiological findings and short-term neurological outcome. Neuropediatrics 35: 283–289

12.   Leijser LM et al. (2006) Using cerebral ultrasound effectively in the newborn infant. Early Hum Dev . 82:827–35

13.   Levene MI (2001) The asphyxiated newborn infant. In: Levene MI et al. (eds) Fetal and neonatal neurology and neurosurgery. Churchill Livingstone, London

14.   Levene MI, De Vries LS (2001) Neonatal intracranial hemorrhage. In: Levene MI et al. (eds) Fetal and neonatal neurology and neurosurgery. Churchill Livingstone, London

15.   Levene MI et al. (1985) Ultrasound of the infant brain, 1st edn. Blackwell Scientific Publications, Oxford

16.   Lorenz JM, Paneth N (2000) Treatment decisions for the extremely premature infant. J Pediatr 137: 593–595

17.   Murphy DJ et al. (1996) Ultrasound findings and clinical antecedents of cerebral palsy in very preterm infants. Arch Dis Child Fetal Neonatal Ed 74: F105–F109

18.   Murphy NP et al. (1989) Cranial ultrasound assessment of gestational age in low birthweight infants. Arch Dis Child 64: 569–572

19.   Naidich TP et al. (1994) The developing cerebral surface. Preliminary report on the patterns of sulcal and gyral maturation – anatomy, ultrasound, and magnetic resonance imaging. Neuroimaging Clin N Am 4: 201–240

20.   van Wezel-Meijler G et al. (1998) Magnetic resonance imaging of the brain in premature infants during the neonatal period. Normal phenomena and reflection of mild ultrasound abnormalities. Neuropediatrics 29: 89–96

21.   van Wezel-Meijler G et al. (1999a) Unilateral thalamic lesions in premature infants: risk factors and short-term prognosis. Neuropediatrics 30: 300–306

22. van Wezel-Meijler G et al. (1999b) Predictive value of neonatal MRI as compared to ultrasound in premature infants with mild periventricular white matter changes. Neuropediatrics 30: 231–238

23. Vollmer B et al. (2003) Predictors of long-term outcome in very preterm infants: gestational age versus neonatal cranial ultrasound. Pediatrics 112: 1108–1114

24. Vollmer B et al. (2006) Long-term neurodevelopmental outcome of preterm children with unilateral cerebral lesions diagnosed by neonatal ultrasound. Early Hum 82:655–61

25. Volpe JJ (2001a) Bacterial and fungal intracranial infections. In: Volpe JJ (ed) Neurology of the newborn. WB Saunders, Philadelphia

26. Volpe JJ (2001b) Hypoxic-ischemic encephalopathy: clinical aspects. In: Volpe JJ (ed) Neurology of the newborn. WB Saunders, Philadelphia

27. Volpe JJ (2001c) Intracranial hemorrhage: germinal matrix-intraventricular hemorrhage of the premature infant. In: Volpe JJ (ed) Neurology of the newborn. WB Saunders, Philadelphia

28. Volpe JJ (2001d) Intracranial hemorrhage: subdural, primary subaracnoid, intracerebellar, intraventricular (term infant), and miscellaneous. In: Volpe JJ (ed) Neurology of the newborn. WB Saunders, Philadelphia

29. Volpe JJ (2001e) Viral, protozoan, and related intracranial infections. In: Volpe JJ (ed) Neurology of the newborn. WB Saunders, Philadelphia

Cranial Ultrasonography: Technical Aspects

For good-quality and safe CUS the following conditions need to be fulfilled: a high-quality modern ultrasound machine with appropriate transducers to enable optimal image quality, and an experienced sonographer who is aware of the special needs of sick newborn and/or preterm infants.

2.1 Equipment

2.1.1 Ultrasound Machine

The ultrasound machine should be a transportable real-time scanner, allowing bedside examinations without the need to transport the baby *(see Fig. 1.1)*. It should be equipped with appropriate transducers, special software for CUS and colour Doppler flow measurements, and a storage system. Facilities for direct printing of images may be useful. Settings need to be optimised for neonatal brain imaging. It is recommended that special CUS presets be used; these can be installed by the application specialist. In individual cases and under certain circumstances, the settings can be adjusted.

2.1.2 Transducers

The use of sector or curved linear array transducers is recommended. High-frequency transducers have high near-field resolution (the higher the transducer frequency, the better the resolution), but they do not allow the same penetration as lower-frequency transducers. The ultrasound system should therefore be equipped with a multifrequency transducer (5–7.5–10 MHz) or different frequency transducers (5, 7.5, and 10 MHz). The transducers should be appropriately sized for an almost perfect fit on the anterior fontanel *(Fig. 2.1)*. To allow good contact between the transducer and the skin, transducer gel is used. In most cases, especially in preterm infants, the distance between the transducer and the brain is small, allowing the use of high-frequency transducers. In most circumstances, good images can be obtained using a transducer frequency of around 7.5 MHz. This enables optimal visualisation of the peri- and intraventricular areas of the brain. For the evaluation of more superficial structures (cortex, subcortical white matter, subarachnoid spaces, superior sagittal sinus) and/or in very tiny infants with small heads, it is advised to perform an additional scan, using a higher frequency up to

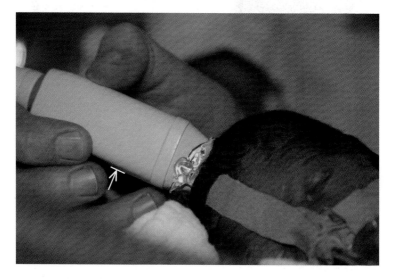

Fig. 2.1 Well-fitting ultrasound probe, positioned onto the anterior fontanel. *Arrow* indicates the marker on the probe

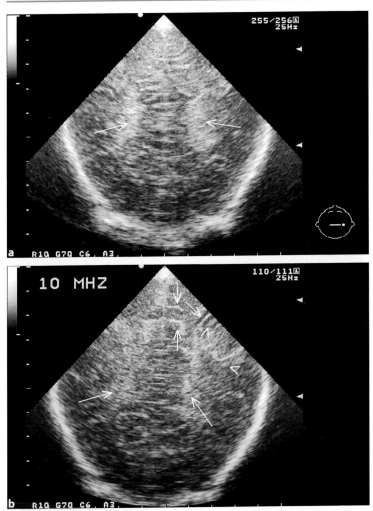

Fig. 2.2 a Coronal ultrasound scan at the level of the parieto-occipital lobes in a full-term baby, born asphyxiated, using a transducer frequency of 7.5 MHz. **b** Coronal ultrasound scan in the same baby at the same level after increasing the transducer frequency up to 10 MHz, now showing more details of the superficial cortical (*short arrows*) and subcortical structures (*arrowheads*). Images show increased echogenicity of the parietal white matter (*arrows*), best seen with the transducer frequency set at 7.5 MHz (**a**), and the subcortical white matter (*arrowheads*), best seen with transducer frequency of 10 MHz (**b**)

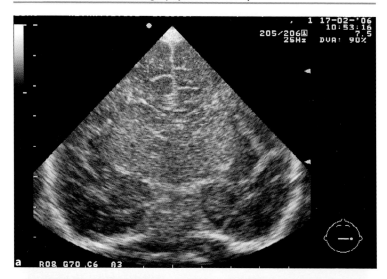

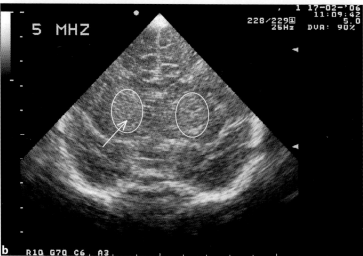

Fig. 2.3 a Coronal ultrasound scan in a full-term baby, born asphyxiated, at the level of the frontal horns of the lateral ventricles. Transducer frequency of 7.5 MHz. **b** Coronal ultrasound scan in the same baby after decreasing the transducer frequency down to 5 MHz, now showing more clearly the subtly increased echogenicity of the basal ganglia (*arrow*). Basal ganglia injury became more obvious during the following days

10 MHz *(Fig. 2.2)*. If deeper penetration of the beam is required, as in larger, older infants or infants with thick, curly hair or in order to obtain a better view of the deeper structures (posterior fossa, basal ganglia in full-term infants), additional scanning with a lower frequency (down to about 5 MHz) is recommended *(Fig. 2.3)*.

2.2   Data Management

Images need to be reproducible. Therefore, it is recommended that a dedicated digital storage system be used, allowing reliable storage and post-imaging assessment. In addition, direct printing of standard views and (suspected) abnormalities can be useful, as it enables storage in the medical files.

2.3   Sonographer and Safety Precautions

The sonographer can be an ultrasound technician or a physician (i.e. ultrasound physician, neuro- or paediatric radiologist, neonatologist). He or she should be specially trained to perform safe, reliable neonatal CUS examinations. In addition, he or she should be well informed with regard to the normal ultrasound anatomy and specific features of the neonatal brain and to the maturational phenomena occurring in the (preterm) neonate's brain. He or she also needs to be well informed about frequently occurring, often (gestational) age-specific brain anomalies (whether congenital or acquired) in the neonate and young infant and be able to recognise these and search for them. The sonographer should also be aware of the special needs of vulnerable, sick (preterm) neonates and should take the necessary hygiene precautions (such as appropriate hand hygiene and cleaning of the ultrasound machine and transducers according to hospital regulations). The transducer gel should be sterile and stored at room temperature. Cooling of the infant due to opening of the incubator needs to be avoided.

CUS Equipment and Procedure	Transducers
• Modern, portable ultrasound machine • Special CUS software • Standard CUS settings; adjust when necessary • Digital storage system • Printed copies • Avoid manipulation and cooling of infant • Take necessary hygiene precautions	• 5–7.5–10 MHz • Appropriately sized • Standard examination: use 7.5–8 MHz • Tiny infant and/or superficial structures: use additional higher frequency (10 MHz) • Large infant, thick hair, and/or deep structures: use additional lower frequency (5 MHz)

Further Reading

1.   American Institute of Ultrasound in Medicine (2006) Standards for performance of the ultrasound examination of the infant brain. www.aium.com

3.   Couture A (2001) Anoxic-ischemic cerebral damage. In: Couture A, Veyrac C (eds) Transfontanellar Doppler imaging in neonates. Springer, Berlin

4.   Couture A et al. (1987) New imaging of cerebral ischemic lesions. High frequency probes and pulsed Doppler. Ann Radiol 30:452–461

5.   De Vries LS, Groenendaal F (2002) Neuroimaging in the preterm infant. Ment Retard Dev Disabil Res Rev 8:273–280

6.   De Vries LS et al. (1992) The spectrum of leukomalacia using cranial ultrasound. Behav Brain Res 49:1–6

10.   Govaert P, De Vries LS (1997) An atlas of neonatal brain sonography. MacKeith Press, Cambridge

11.   Leijser LM et al. (2004) Hyperechogenicity of the thalamus and basal ganglia in very preterm infants: radiological findings and short-term neurological outcome. Neuropediatrics 35:283–289

12.   Levene MI (2001a) The asphyxiated newborn infant. In: Levene MI et al. (eds) Fetal and neonatal neurology and neurosurgery. Churchill Livingstone, London

13.   Levene MI, De Vries LS (2001b) Neonatal intracranial hemorrhage. In: Levene MI et al. (eds) Fetal and neonatal neurology and neurosurgery. Churchill Livingstone, London

15. Naidich TP et al. (1994) The developing cerebral surface. Preliminary report on the patterns of sulcal and gyral maturation – anatomy, ultrasound, and magnetic resonance imaging. Neuroimaging Clin N Am 4:201–240

16. Van Wezel-Meijler G et al. (1998) Magnetic resonance imaging of the brain in premature infants during the neonatal period. Normal phenomena and reflection of mild ultrasound abnormalities. Neuropediatrics 29:89–96

17. Veyrac C et al. (2006) Brain ultrasonography in the premature infant. Pediatr Radiol 36:626–635

18. Volpe JJ (2001a) Hypoxic-ischemic encephalopathy: clinical aspects. In: Volpe JJ (ed) Neurology of the newborn. WB Saunders, Philadelphia

19. Volpe JJ (2001b) Intracranial hemorrhage: germinal matrix-intraventricular hemorrhage of the premature infant. In: Volpe JJ (ed) Neurology of the newborn. WB Saunders, Philadelphia

20. Volpe JJ (2001c) Intracranial hemorrhage: subdural, primary subarachnoid, intracerebellar, intraventricular (term infant), and miscellaneous. In: Volpe JJ (ed) Neurology of the newborn. WB Saunders, Philadelphia

3

Performing Cranial Ultrasound Examinations

Preterm infants and sick full-term infants are examined in their incubator while maintaining monitoring of vital functions *(see also Chap. 2 and Fig. 1.1)*. It is recommended that the CUS examination be performed while only the incubator windows are open. Manipulation of the infant (with the exception of minor adjustments) is rarely necessary while scanning through the anterior fontanel. Older infants and full-term, well neonates can be examined in their cot or car seat or on an adult's lap *(Fig. 3.1)*.

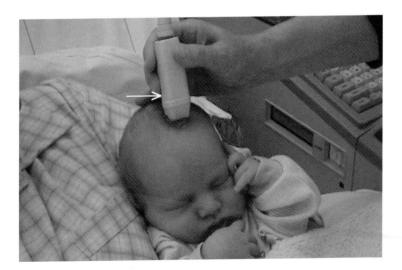

Fig. 3.1 Ultrasound examination performed in a full-term newborn infant while infant is seated on his mother's lap (*arrow* indicates marker on probe)

3.1   Standard Views

For a standard CUS procedure to enable optimal visualisation of the supratentorial structures, the anterior fontanel is used as an acoustic window. Images are recorded in at least six standard coronal and five standard sagittal planes. These standard planes and the anatomical structures visualised in these planes are presented in Part II.

In addition to the standard planes, the whole brain should be scanned to obtain an overview of the brain's appearance. This allows assessment of the anatomical structures and detection of subtle changes and small and/or superficially located lesions. Besides the standard views, for any suspected abnormality, images should be recorded in two planes *(Fig. 3.2)*.

3.1.1   Coronal Planes

The anterior fontanel is palpated and the transducer is positioned in the middle, with the marker on the probe turned to the right side of the baby *(see Fig. 2.1)*. The left side of the brain will thus be projected on the right side of the monitor, and vice versa *(Fig. 3.3)*. The probe is subsequently angled sufficiently far forwards and backwards to scan the entire brain from the frontal lobes at the level of the orbits to the occipital lobes *(see Part II)*.

3.1.2   Sagittal Planes

The transducer is again positioned in the middle of the anterior fontanel, and the marker is now pointing towards the baby's mid-face *(Fig. 3.4)*. The anterior part of the brain will thus be projected on the left side of the monitor *(Fig. 3.5)*. First, a good view of the midline is obtained. The transducer is subsequently angled sufficiently to the right and the left to scan out to the Sylvian fissures and insulae on both sides *(see Part II)*. Because the lateral ventricles fan out posteriorly, the transducer should be positioned slightly slanting, with the back part of the transducer slightly

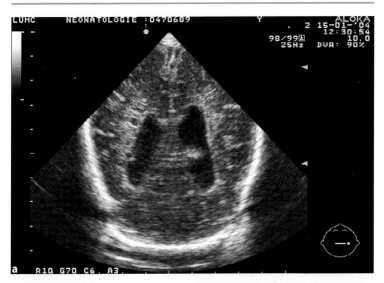

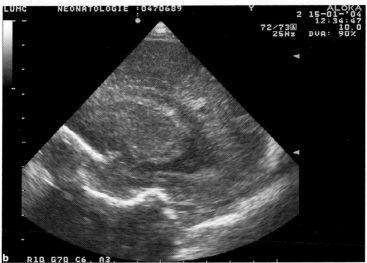

Fig. 3.2a,b Ultrasound scan in a preterm infant with cystic periventricular leukomalacia, showing cystic lesions and increased echogenicity in the parietal periventricular white matter, seen in two image directions. **a** Coronal scan at the level of the trigone of the lateral ventricles. **b** Parasagittal scan through the right lateral ventricle

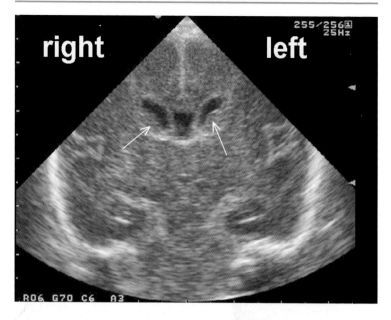

Fig. 3.3 Coronal ultrasound scan in a very preterm infant at the level of the frontal horns of the lateral ventricles. If the marker on the transducer is positioned in the right corner of the anterior fontanel *(see Figs. 2.1 and 3.1)*, the right side of the brain is projected on the left side of the image, and vice versa. Image shows germinal matrix haemorrhages of older duration *(arrows)*

more lateral than the front part. While the second or fourth parasagittal planes are being obtained, this enables visualisation of the lateral ventricle over its entire length *(see Fig. 3.5 and Part II)*.

When scanning in the sagittal planes, it is important to mark which side of the brain is being scanned. This can either be done using the body marker application or by an annotation *(Fig. 3.6)*.

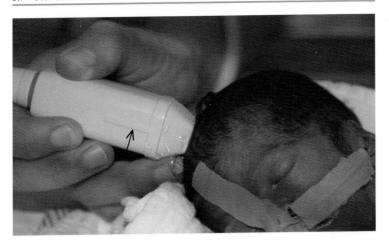

Fig. 3.4 Probe positioning for obtaining parasagittal scan. *Arrow* indicates marker

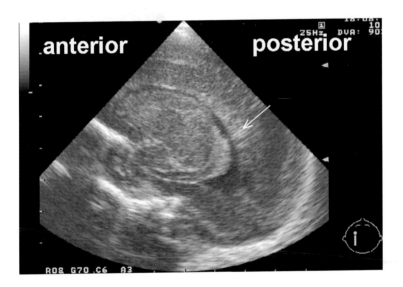

Fig. 3.5 Parasagittal ultrasound scan in a preterm infant through the left lateral ventricle. If the marker on the transducer is pointing towards the baby's nose *(see Fig. 3.4),* the anterior part of the brain will be projected on the left of the image and the posterior part on the right. Image shows some increased echogenicity in the parietal periventricular white matter *(arrow)*

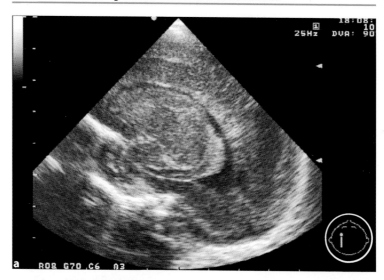

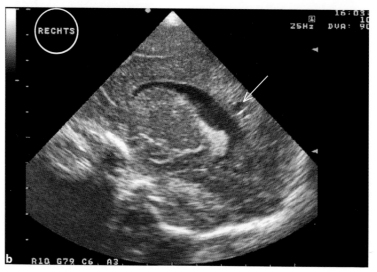

Fig. 3.6a,b Using markers. **a** Parasagittal ultrasound scan through the left lateral ventricle as is shown by the body marker (*same image as Fig. 3.5*). **b** Parasagittal ultrasound scan through the right lateral ventricle, as is annotated. Image shows cystic lesions in the parietal region (*arrow*) and a dilated lateral ventricle (grade 2 PVL)

3.2 Supplemental Acoustic Windows

If only the anterior fontanel is used as an acoustic window, brain structures further away from this fontanel cannot be visualised with high-frequency transducers. Lower frequencies enable deeper penetration *(see Fig. 2.2)*, but detailed information is lost. Better visualisation can be obtained using acoustic windows closer to these structures, thus allowing the use of higher-frequency, high-resolution transducers and visualisation from different angles *(Fig. 3.7)*.

Using these supplemental acoustic windows for CUS examinations requires additional skills, practice, and anatomical knowledge. The views thus obtained and the anatomical structures visualised will be presented

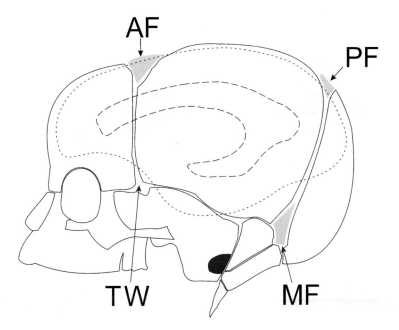

Fig. 3.7 The acoustic windows. *AF* anterior fontanel, *PF* posterior fontanel, *MF* mastoid (or postero-lateral) fontanel, *TW* temporal window

in Part II. In order to avoid excessive manipulation of the infant, it is recommended to apply only those acoustic windows that are easily accessible (i.e. if the infant is positioned on his or her left side, only the right-sided windows are used, and vice versa). The examination can be continued when the infant is in another position.

Indications for CUS using supplemental windows are presented in *Appendix 3.1*

3.2.1   Posterior Fontanel

The posterior fontanel, located between the parietal and occipital bones *(see Fig. 3.7)*, enables a good view of the occipital horns of the lateral

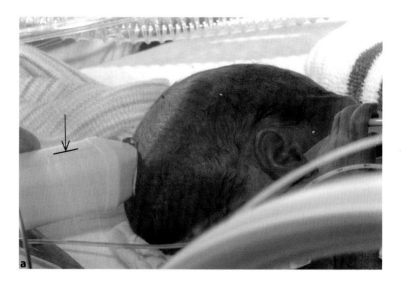

Fig. 3.8a,b Posterior fontanel. **a** Probe positioning for coronal scan using the posterior fontanel as an acoustic window (*arrow* indicates marker). **b** *see next page*

ventricles, the occipital parenchyma, and the posterior fossa structures. Using this fontanel, scanning can be done in the coronal and sagittal planes. The posterior fontanel is palpated and the transducer placed in the middle of the fontanel, with the marker in the horizontal position to obtain a coronal plane and in the vertical position to obtain a sagittal plane *(Fig. 3.8)*. Scanning through the posterior fontanel enables more accurate detection of blood in the occipital horns of the lateral ventricles, injury to the occipital white matter or cortex, cerebellar haemorrhage, and posterior fossa malformations *(Figs. 3.9, 3.10)*

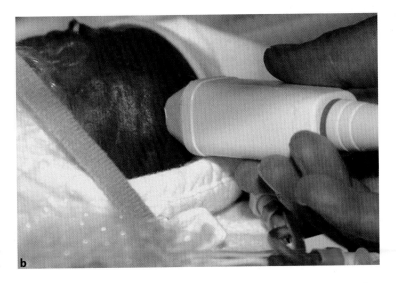

Fig. 3.8 *(continued)* **b** Probe positioning for parasagittal scan using the posterior fontanel as an acoustic window. The marker (not shown here) is on the top of the probe, pointing towards the cranium

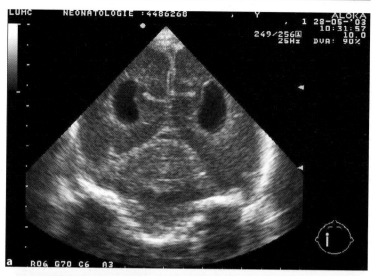

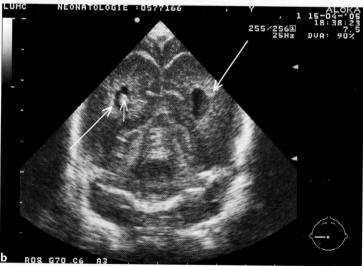

Fig. 3.9a–c Coronal ultrasound scans obtained through the posterior fontanel in very preterm infants. **a** Normal. **b** Increased echogenicity in the occipital white matter (*arrows*) and a blood clot in the occipital horn of the lateral ventricle (*short arrow*). **c** *see next page*

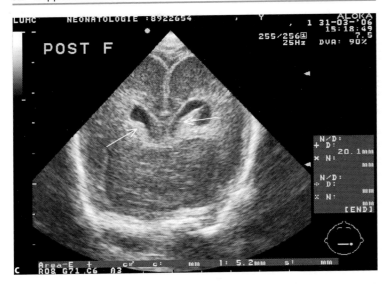

Fig. 3.9 *(continued)* **c** Intraventricular haemorrhage with blood clots in the occipital horns of the left lateral ventricle (*arrows*)

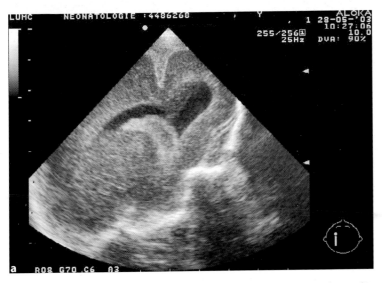

Fig. 3.10a,b Parasagittal ultrasound scans obtained through the posterior fontanel in a very preterm infant. **a** Normal. **b** *see next page*

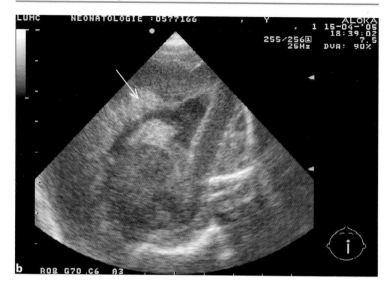

Fig. 3.10 (continued) **b** Increased echogenicity in the periventricular white matter (arrow) (Same patient as in Fig. 3.9b)

3.2.2   Temporal Windows

Good transverse views of the brain stem can be obtained through the temporal window. The transducer is placed above the ear, approximately 1 cm above and anterior to the external auditory meatus, with the marker in a horizontal position. The transducer position is subsequently adjusted until visualisation of the brain stem is obtained (Fig. 3.11). The image quality in this view depends on the bony thickness. Scanning through the temporal window allows Doppler flow measurements in the circle of Willis and detection of brain stem and cerebellar haemorrhages (Fig. 3.12).

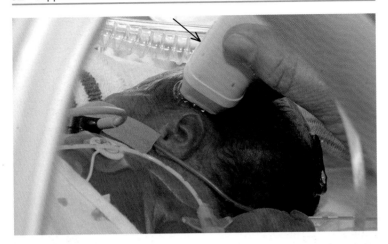

Fig. 3.11 Temporal window. Probe positioning for CUS using temporal window, providing transverse views (*arrow* indicates marker)

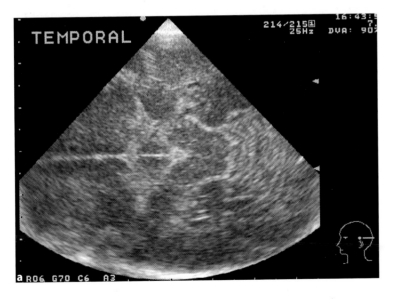

Fig. 3.12a,b Temporal window. **a** Normal transverse view of brain stem and upper cerebellum, obtained through temporal window. **b** *see next page*

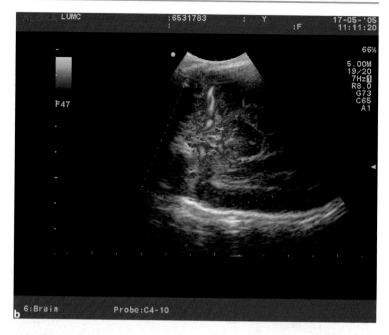

Fig. 3.12 *(continued)* **b** Transverse view of brain stem showing circle of Willis, using colour Doppler

3.2.3   Mastoid Fontanels

The mastoid fontanels are located at the junction of the temporal, occipital, and posterior parietal bones *(see Fig. 3.7).* These windows allow visualisation of the posterior fossa and the midbrain in two planes, thus enabling detection of congenital anomalies and haemorrhages in these areas, in particular cerebellar haemorrhages and dilatation of the third and fourth ventricles *(Fig. 3.13).* After the auricle is gently bent forward, the transducer is placed behind the ear, just above the tragus, and subsequently moved until a good view of the posterior fossa is obtained. If the transducer is positioned with the marker in a vertical direction, a coronal plane is obtained. If the marker is in a horizontal position, a transverse view is obtained *(Fig. 3.14).*

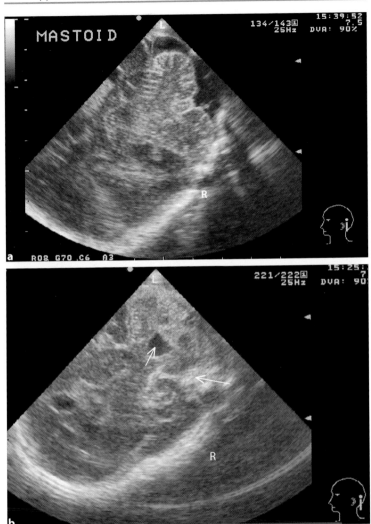

Fig. 3.13a,b Mastoid fontanel. **a** Coronal view through the left mastoid fontanel in a preterm baby, showing a normal cerebellum. **b** Coronal view through the left lateral ventricle in a preterm baby, with the transducer positioned more anteriorly, showing irregular increased echogenicity in the right cerebellar hemisphere (*arrow*), diagnosed as cerebellar haemorrhage (confirmed by MRI) and a wide fourth ventricle (*short arrow*). *R* right, *L* left

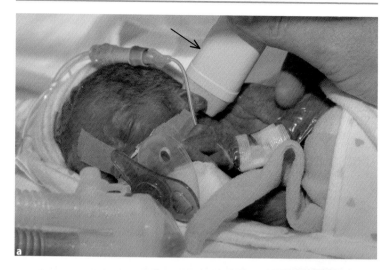

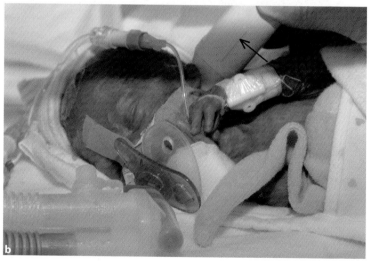

Fig. 3.14a,b Mastoid fontanel. **a** Probe position for coronal view using the mastoid fontanel as an acoustic window. **b** Probe position for transverse view using the mastoid fontanel as an acoustic window. *Arrows* indicate marker on probe

3.3   Doppler Flow Measurements

(Colour) Doppler ultrasonography can be applied to study cerebral haemodynamics. Blood flow velocity can be measured in the major cerebral arteries and their branches and in the basilar and internal carotid arteries *(see Fig. 3.12b)* and the large veins (i.e. internal cerebral veins, vein of Galen, superior sagittal, straight and transverse sinus). Doppler flow measurements may help to distinguish between vascular structures and non-vascular lesions. Blood flow velocities in the major cerebral arteries can be of prognostic significance in infants with hypoxic-ischaemic cerebral damage.

A detailed overview of the role of cerebral Doppler imaging is provided in the recent book by Couture and Veyrac *(2001)*.

Standard CUS procedure	Supplemental acoustic windows
• Anterior fontanel = acoustic window (supratentorial structures) • Scan whole brain from frontal to occipital and right to left • Record at least six standard coronal and five standard (para)sagittal planes • Record (suspected) abnormalities in two planes	• Posterior fontanel (occipital parenchyma, occipital horns, posterior fossa) • Mastoid fontanels (midbrain, posterior fossa, ventricular system) • Temporal windows (midbrain, circle of Willis, flow measurements)

Appendix 3.1   Indications for Scanning Through Supplemental Windows

- Preterm, gestational age < 30 weeks, around third day (cerebellar haemorrhage?)
- Preterm, complicated medical course with circulatory and/or respiratory instability

- Peri- and intraventricular haemorrhage (blood in occipital horns? Concomitant cerebellar haemorrhage?)
- Suspected posterior fossa haemorrhage on standard CUS
- Suspected posterior fossa abnormalities
- Ventricular dilatation of unknown cause

Reference

1.   Couture A, Veyrac C (2001) Transfontanellar Doppler imaging in neonates, 1st edn. Springer, Berlin

Further Reading

1.   Anderson N et al. (1994) Diagnosis of intraventricular hemorrhage in the newborn: value of sonography via the posterior fontanelle. AJR Am J Roentgenol 163:893–896

2.   Anderson NG et al. (1995) Posterior fontanelle cranial ultrasound: anatomic and sonographic correlation. Early Hum Dev 42:141–152

3.   Buckley KM et al. (1997) Use of the mastoid fontanelle for improved sonographic visualization of the neonatal midbrain and posterior fossa. AJR Am J Roentgenol 168:1021–1025

4.   Correa F et al. (2004) Posterior fontanelle sonography: an acoustic window into the neonatal brain. AJNR Am J Neuroradiol 25:1274–1282

5.   Couture A et al. (2001) Advanced cranial ultrasound: transfontanellar Doppler imaging in neonates. Eur Radiol 11:2399–2410

6.   Dean LM, Taylor GA (1995) The intracranial venous system in infants: normal and abnormal findings on duplex and color Doppler sonography. AJR Am J Roentgenol 164:151–156

7.   Di Salvo DN (2001) A new view of the neonatal brain: clinical utility of supplemental neurologic US imaging windows. Radiographics 21:943–955

8.   Kilby M et al. (2001) Doppler assessment of the fetal and neonatal brain. In: Levene MI et al. (eds) Fetal and neonatal neurology and neurosurgery. Churchill Livingstone, London

9. Luna JA, Goldstein RB (2000) Sonographic visualization of neonatal posterior fossa abnormalities through the posterolateral fontanelle. AJR Am J Roentgenol 174:561–567

10. Taylor GA (1992) Intracranial venous system in the newborn: evaluation of normal anatomy and flow characteristics with color Doppler US. Radiology 183:449–452

11. Taylor GA (2001) Sonographic assessment of posthemorrhagic ventricular dilatation. Radiol Clin North Am 39:541–551

12. Van Bel F et al. (1993) Changes in cerebral hemodynamics and oxygenation in the first 24 hours after birth asphyxia. Pediatrics 92:365–372

13. Veyrac C et al. (2006) Brain ultrasonography in the premature infant. Pediatr Radiol 36:626–635

14. Yousefzadeh DK, Naidich TP (1985) US anatomy of the posterior fossa in children: correlation with brain sections. Radiology 156:353–361

4 Assessing Cranial Ultrasound Examinations

4.1 Assessing Cranial Ultrasound Examinations

When performing and assessing CUS examinations, the **anatomy** *(see Part II)* and **maturation** *(see Chap. 8)* of the brain are evaluated, and signs of **pathology**, whether congenital or acquired, are sought. In general, cerebral anomalies or injury should be visualised in at least two different planes *(see Fig. 3.2)*. An overview of cerebral pathology as can be visualised by CUS is provided in the *Atlas on Cranial Ultrasonography* by Govaert and De Vries *(1997)*.

4.1.1 A Systematic Approach to Detect Cerebral Pathology

While looking for signs of pathology, a systematic approach is recommended. The following can be used as a guideline:

- Are the **anatomical** structures distinguishable, and do they appear normal? *(See Part II; Fig. 4.1)*
- Does the **maturation** of the brain (cortical folding) appear appropriate for GA? *(See Chap. 8; Fig. 4.2)*
- Is there a normal distinction between the cortex and the white matter? *(Fig. 4.3)*
- Is the echogenicity of the cortical grey matter normal? *(Fig. 4.4)*
- Is there normal echogenicity and homogeneity of the periventricular and subcortical white matter? *(Fig. 4.5)*
- Is there normal echogenicity and homogeneity of the thalami and basal ganglia? *(Fig. 4.6)*

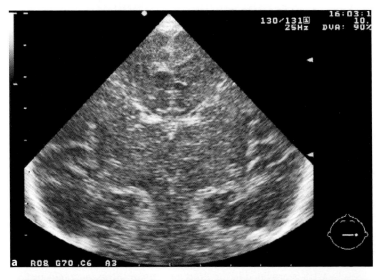

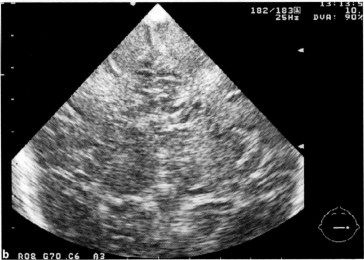

Fig. 4.1a,b Coronal ultrasound scan at the level of the bodies of the lateral ventricles. **a** Normal image in a full-term neonate. **b** Loss of normal architecture and diffusely increased echogenicity in a full-term neonate with severe hypoxic-ischaemic brain damage

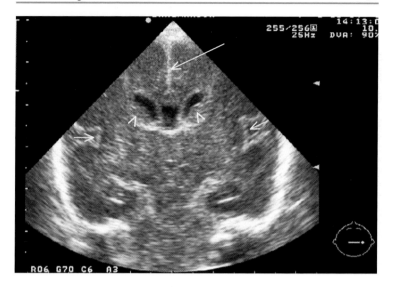

Fig. 4.2 Coronal ultrasound scan at the level of the bodies of the lateral ventricles in a preterm infant (GA 26 weeks), showing smooth interhemispheric fissure (*arrow*) and wide open Sylvian fissures (*short arrows*). Also shows bilateral germinal matrix haemorrhage of longer duration (*arrowheads*). Brain maturation appropriate for GA. Compare image with Fig. 4.1a

- Do the size, width, lining and echogenicity of the ventricular system appear normal? *(Figs. 4.7 and 4.8)*
- In the case of ventricular enlargement, are the lateral ventricles measured according to standard guidelines? *(Fig. 4.8) (Levene 1981, Davies et al. 2000; see also Appendix 4.1 and Figs. 4.11 and 4.12)*
- Are the widths of the subarachnoid spaces appropriate for age? *(Fig. 4.9)*
- Is there a midline shift? *(Fig. 4.10)*

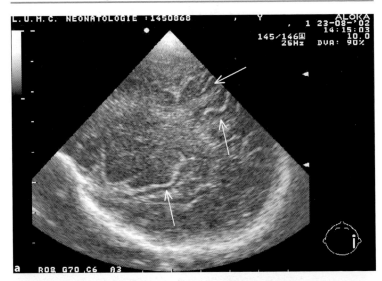

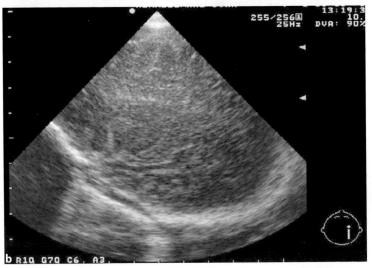

Fig. 4.3a,b Parasagittal ultrasound scan through the insula. **a** Normal image in a full-term neonate, showing normal hypo-echogenic cortex (*arrows*) and distinction between cortex and white matter. **b** Loss of normal grey–white matter differentiation with blurring of the cortex in a full-term neonate with hypoxic-ischaemic brain injury

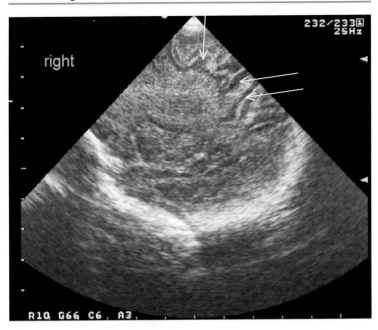

Fig. 4.4 Parasagittal ultrasound scan through the insula in a full-term baby with widespread hypoxic-ischaemic cortical and subcortical damage, showing a widened hypoechogenic cortex (*arrows*). Compare image with normal image of Fig. 4.3a

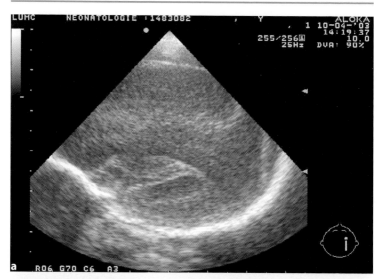

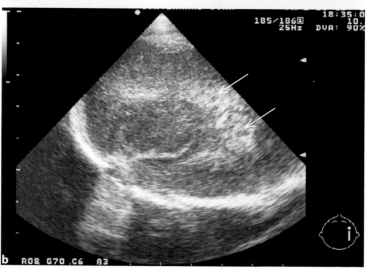

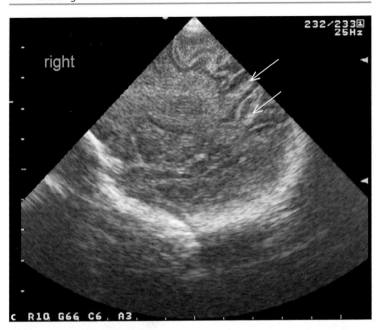

Fig. 4.5a–c Parasagittal ultrasound scan through the insula. **a** Preterm infant (GA 26 weeks), showing normal echogenicity of the periventricular white matter. Also shows very smooth, unfolded cortex. Same infant as in Fig. 4.2. **b** Preterm infant (GA 29 weeks), showing inhomogeneously increased echogenicity of the periventricular white matter (*arrows*), so-called periventricular "flaring." **c** Full-term infant with widespread hypoxic-ischaemic cortical and subcortical damage (same image as Fig. 4.4), showing increased echogenicity of the subcortical white matter (*arrows*). Compare image with normal image of Fig. 4.3a

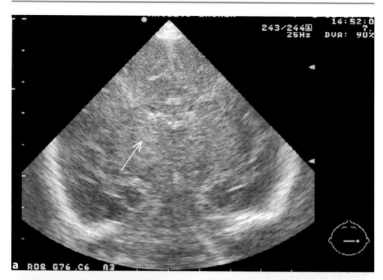

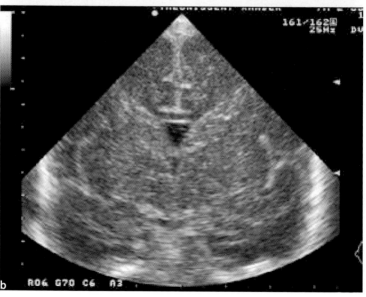

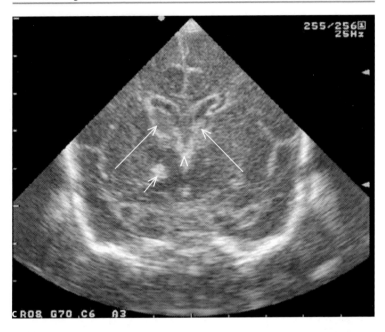

Fig. 4.6a–c Coronal ultrasound scan at the level of the bodies of the lateral ventricles. **a** Full-term infant with hypoxic-ischaemic cerebral damage, showing increased echogenicity of the basal ganglia and thalami, being most pronounced on the right side (*arrows*) and having a "fuzzy" appearance with loss of normal architecture. Compare with normal image in Fig. 4.1a. **b** Preterm infant (GA 31 weeks), showing normal basal ganglia (level of the image is slightly more frontal than in **a** and **c**). **c** Preterm baby (GA 33 weeks) with bilateral intraventricular haemorrhage (*arrows*) of longer duration and blood clot in the third ventricle (*arrowhead*), showing local echodensity in the basal ganglia on the right side (*short arrow*)

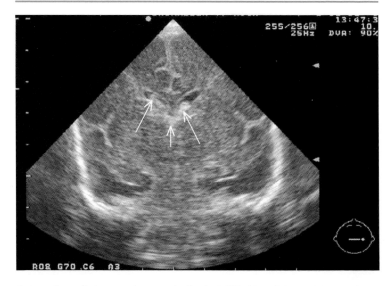

Fig. 4.7 Coronal ultrasound scan at the level of the bodies of the lateral ventricles in a preterm infant (GA 30 weeks), showing bilateral (*arrows*) with blood clot in the third ventricle (*short arrow*). Compare with normal image in Fig. 4.6b

▷ **Fig. 4.8a,b** Coronal ultrasound scan at the level of the bodies of the lateral ventricles. **a** Preterm infant (GA 31 weeks) showing bilateral IVH (*arrows*) with ventricular dilatation, echodense ventricular lining (*arrowhead*), and widened third ventricle (*short arrow*). Also showing dilated temporal horns of the lateral ventricles (*long arrows*). Ventricular index is measured according to Levene (the indicated distance to be divided by 2) *(1981)*. **b** Preterm infant (GA 29 weeks), showing bilateral IVH (*arrows*) with asymmetric ventricular dilatation. Also shows right-sided periventricular haemorrhagic infarction (*short arrow*) and echodensity in the basal ganglia (*arrowhead*). The anterior horn width is measured according to Davies et al. *(2000)*. Compare with normal image in Fig. 4.6b (level of the image in Fig. 4.6b is slightly more frontal)

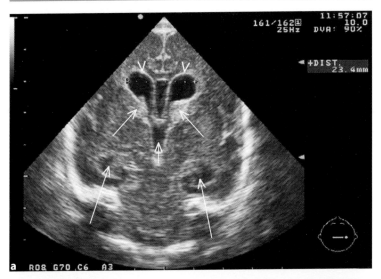

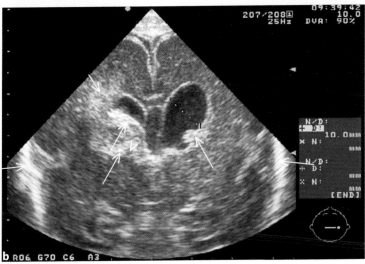

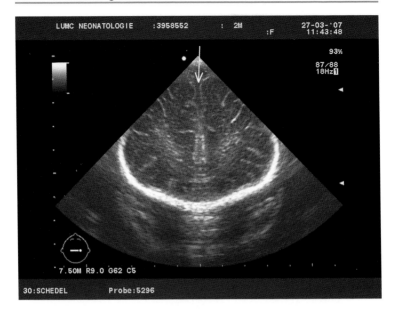

Fig. 4.9 Coronal ultrasound scan at the level of the frontal lobes in a very preterm infant scanned at term age, showing wide subarachnoid space (*arrow*)

Image assessment

- Anatomy
- Maturation
- Distinction of cortex/white matter
- Echogenicity of cortex
- Echogenicity/homogeneity of white matter
- Echogenicity/homogeneity of deep grey matter
- Ventricular system: size, lining, echogenicity
  if dilated: perform serial measurements
- Width of subarachnoid spaces
- Midline shift

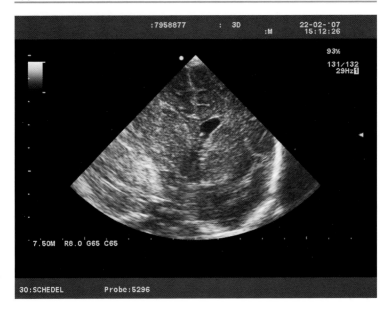

Fig. 4.10 Coronal ultrasound scan in a full-term neonate (level of the frontal horns of the lateral ventricles), showing midline shift, increased echogenicity in the right temporal region, and compressed frontal horn of the right lateral ventricle due to massive haemorrhage in the right temporal lobe

Appendix 4.1   Measurement of the Lateral Ventricles

- In the third coronal plane (at the level of the interventricular foramina of Monro), the "ventricular index" is measured as the largest distance in millimetres between the frontal horns. This number, if divided by 2, results in the "ventricular index" (VI), according to Levene. Normal values are available *(Fig. 4.11; see also Fig. 4.8a).* [Adapted from Levene (1981)]
- According to Davies (2000), the width of the anterior horn of the lateral ventricles is measured in the third coronal plane (at the level of the interventricular foramina of Monro). The width is measured on each side as the distance between the medial wall and the floor of the lateral ventricle at the widest point *(Fig. 4.12; see also Fig. 4.8b)*

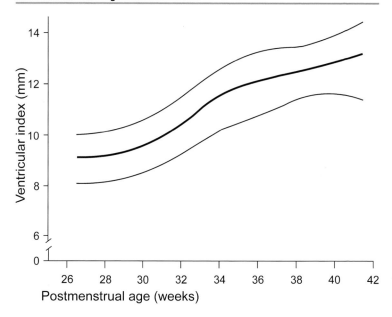

Fig. 4.11 Growth charts of the ventricular index according to Levene *(1981) (see also Appendix 4.1)*. Reproduced with permission from BMJ Publishing Group

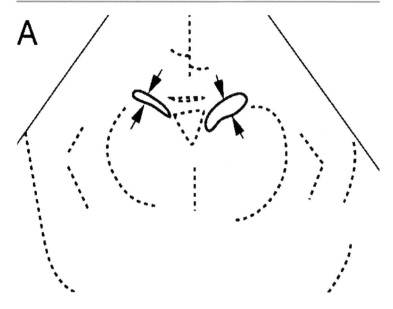

Fig. 4.12 Measurement of anterior horn width, according to Davies et al. *(2000) (see also Appendix 4.1).* Reproduced with permission from BMJ Publishing Group

References

1.   Davies MW et al. (2000) Reference ranges for the linear dimensions of the intracranial ventricles in preterm neonates. Arch Dis Child Fetal Neonatal Ed 82: F218–F223
2.   Govaert P, De Vries LS (1997) An atlas of neonatal brain sonography, 1st edn. MacKeith Press, Cambridge
3.   Levene MI (1981) Measurement of the growth of the lateral ventricles in preterm infants with real-time ultrasound. Arch Dis Child 56:900–904

Further Reading

1.   Arthur R, Ramenghi L (2001a) Imaging the neonatal brain. In: Levene MI et al. (eds) Fetal and neonatal neurology and neurosurgery. Churchill Livingstone, London

2.   Ashwal S (2001b) Congenital structural defects of the brain. In: Levene MI et al. (eds) Fetal and neonatal neurology and neurosurgery. Churchill Livingstone, London

3.   Lam WW et al. (2001) Ultrasonographic measurement of subarachnoid space in normal infants and children. Pediatr Neurol 25:380–384

4.   Larroche J-C (1987) Le developpement du cerveau foetal humain. Atlas anatomique. INSERM CNRS, Paris

5.   Levene MI (2001c) The asphyxiated newborn infant. In: Levene MI et al. (eds) Fetal and neonatal neurology and neurosurgery. Churchill Livingstone, London

6.   Levene MI, De Vries LS (2001d) Neonatal intracranial hemorrhage. In: Levene MI et al. (eds) Fetal and neonatal neurology and neurosurgery. Churchill Livingstone, London

7.   Libicher M, Troger J (1992) US measurement of the subarachnoid space in infants: normal values. Radiology 184:749–751

8.   Murphy NP et al. (1989) Cranial ultrasound assessment of gestational age in low birthweight infants. Arch Dis Child 64:569–572

9.   Naidich TP et al. (1994) The developing cerebral surface. Preliminary report on the patterns of sulcal and gyral maturation – anatomy, ultrasound, and magnetic resonance imaging. Neuroimaging Clin N Am 4:201–240

10.   Volpe JJ (2001a) Bacterial and fungal intracranial infections. In: Volpe JJ (ed) Neurology of the newborn. WB Saunders, Philadelphia

11.   Volpe JJ (2001b) Hypoxic-ischaemic encephalopathy: clinical aspects. In: Volpe JJ (ed) Neurology of the newborn. WB Saunders, Philadelphia

12.   Volpe JJ (2001c) Intracranial hemorrhage: germinal matrix-intraventricular hemorrhage of the premature infant. In: Volpe JJ (ed) Neurology of the newborn. WB Saunders, Philadelphia

13.   Volpe JJ (2001d) Intracranial hemorrhage: subdural, primary subarachnoid, intracerebellar, intraventricular (term infant), and miscellaneous. In: Volpe JJ (ed) Neurology of the newborn. WB Saunders, Philadelphia

14.   Volpe JJ (2001e) Viral, protozoan, and related intracranial infections. In: Volpe JJ (ed) Neurology of the newborn. WB Saunders, Philadelphia

Timing of Ultrasound Examinations

5.1 Timing of Ultrasound Examinations

In order to obtain optimal prognostic information from CUS serial, carefully timed examinations are essential, both in preterm and sick full-term infants. If timing is not optimally chosen, if time intervals between CUS examinations are too long, or if CUS examinations are discontinued too early, important information and/or injury may be overlooked. Adequate outcome prediction will then be unreliable, and an unfavourable outcome may not be predicted. On the other hand, if the quality of CUS is good, timing is carefully chosen, proper transducers are used, and, in the case of preterm birth, serial examinations are continued until term age, most diagnoses will not remain undetected, and the reliability and prognostic value of CUS can be high. Serial CUS examinations are not only essential for accurate and reliable detection of haemorrhagic, ischaemic, and inflammatory brain damage, but they also enable assessment of the onset of injury and the evolution of lesions.

5.1.1 Ultrasound Screening Programme

In neonatal units it is useful to apply general guidelines for CUS examinations *(see Chaps. 3 and 4)* and a CUS screening programme. In *Table 5.1,* an example of a basic screening programme, as applied at our neonatal intensive care unit (NICU), is presented. This screening programme is used for all infants admitted to our unit, who consist mainly of preterm infants, sick full-term neonates, and neonates with congenital malformations. It calls for at least one CUS examination for each infant, regardless of GA, diagnosis, or medical course, and serial CUS examinations for preterm and sick full-term neonates.

This screening programme is based on the following:
- A first CUS examination soon after birth will give information on congenital anomalies of the brain, congenital infections, some metabolic diseases, traumatic brain injury after traumatic delivery, and the antenatal onset of lesions. It can also serve as a baseline and comparison for the next CUS examinations.
- Haemorrhagic lesions usually become visible within hours of the incident.
- Most haemorrhagic lesions in newborn infants develop around birth.
- More than 90% of peri- and intraventricular haemorrhages (P/IVH) develop within the first 3 days of birth.
- Progression of an initial P/IVH usually occurs within 3 to 5 days.

Table 5.1 *CUS screening programme*

NICU and/or <32 weeks GA and/or birth weight <1,500 g	High care and ≥32 weeks GA and ≥1,500 g
<24 h after birth	
On the third day	On the third day
Biweekly until the second week	
Weekly until discharge	Weekly until discharge
Around term[a]	
More frequently in the case of (suspected) abnormalities	More frequently in the case of (suspected) abnormalities

[a] It is recommended that term CUS be performed at the neonatal centre

Thus, a first CUS examination performed soon after birth (within 24 h) and a second examination performed around the third day will enable detection of most haemorrhagic lesions. By performing a third scan around the seventh day, almost all haemorrhages will be detected and their maximum extent identified.

- It takes a variable period of time (hours to days) before ischaemic lesions become visible.
- The first stages of hypoxic-ischaemic brain damage may evolve over a variable period of time (hours to weeks).
- Especially in preterm infants, the first stages and the milder spectrum of hypoxic-ischaemic brain damage may be hard to distinguish from normal (maturational) phenomena occurring in the immature brain *(Fig. 5.1)*.
- In preterm infants ischaemic lesions may develop throughout the neonatal period, related to postnatal events *(see Fig. 5.2a)*.

Thus:

- A CUS examination performed on the first day of life and repeated at least twice during the first week will enable detection of the acute stages of perinatal hypoxic-ischaemic brain injury.
- Sequential CUS examinations are necessary to assess the evolution of ischaemic lesions and to distinguish (mild) pathology from normal (maturational) phenomena.
- In preterm infants, sequential CUS examinations throughout the neonatal period are necessary to exclude later onset of ischaemic lesions.

For infants who were born prematurely and are later transferred from the neonatal referral centre to a local hospital, arrangements need to be made for continuation of CUS examinations. If local facilities are insufficient, it is recommended that CUS examinations be performed at regular intervals at the neonatal centre.

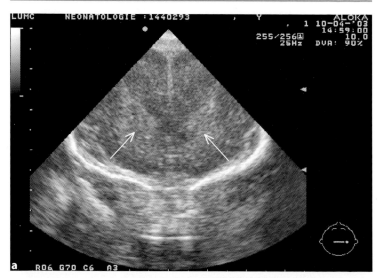

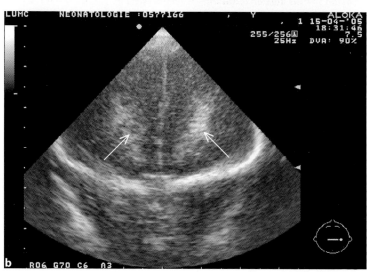

◀ **Fig. 5.1 a** Coronal ultrasound scan at the level of the frontal lobes in a preterm infant (GA 27 weeks), showing symmetrical, bilateral increased echogenicity in the frontal white matter ("frontal echodensities") (*arrows*), which is a normal finding in preterm infants *(van Wezel-Meijler et al. 1998)*. **b** These normal frontal echodensities should not be confused with pathological periventricular flaring (*arrows*): coronal ultrasound scan in a preterm infant, showing asymmetric periventricular flaring in the frontal white matter

5.2   Cranial Ultrasonography at Term Corrected Age

In addition, in infants born very prematurely (GA < 32 weeks) and/or with very low birth weight (< 1,500 g), infants in whom parenchymal injury was demonstrated or suspected, infants at increased risk of brain damage, infants with complicated intraventricular haemorrhage (IVH), and infants with meningitis and/or brain infections, it is recommended that CUS be performed around term age, preferably at the neonatal centre. This term examination is done to see the later stages of (ischaemic) brain injury, to detect new lesions that may have developed after discharge *(Fig. 5.2)*, and to evaluate brain growth and development, which may be impaired in very preterm infants *(see Fig. 4.9)*.

Indications for CUS at term corrected age are presented in *Appendix 5.1*.

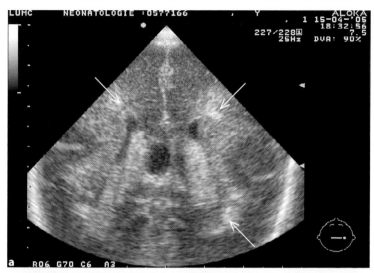

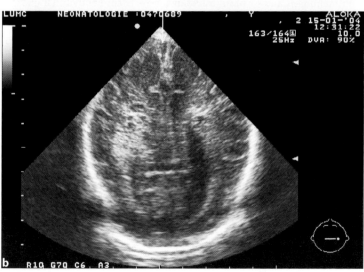

◁ **Fig. 5.2 a** Coronal ultrasound scan at the level of the trigone of the lateral ventricles, showing asymmetric, bilateral periventricular flaring (*arrows*). This preterm infant initially had normal CUS scans but later developed PVL (same infant as in Fig. 5.1b). **b** CUS scan at the level of the parieto-occipital lobes in a preterm infant, imaged at term age. It shows bilateral cystic white matter lesions within hyperechogenic areas. This infant initially had periventricular flaring and developed the cystic lesions after discharge (same infant as in Fig. 4.5b). Also shows wide subarachnoid spaces (*arrow*)

5.3   Adaptations of Ultrasound Examinations, Depending on Diagnosis

When using a CUS screening programme, it is important to realise that such a programme is suitable for neonates without neurological symptoms or brain pathology or for neonates with stable brain abnormalities (such as congenital anomalies or acquired but stabilised lesions). In cases of (suspected) cerebral and/or neurological abnormalities, the intensity and frequency of CUS examinations may need to be increased, depending on the clinical picture and the lesion(s). This can vary between one or two CUS examinations a week in non-progressive cases and several CUS examinations a day in unstable cases (such as IVH and post-haemorrhagic ventricular dilatation (PHVD), severe hypoxic-ischaemic encephalopathy, complicated meningitis, and brain infections).

If complications occur after P/IVH (progression of the haemorrhage, ventricular dilatation, and/or periventricular haemorrhagic infarction) *(see Chap. 6)*, it is recommended that the frequency of CUS examinations be intensified and, in the case of ventricular dilatation, the lateral ventricles be measured on a regular basis until stabilisation has occurred *(see Appendix 4.1, Figs. 4.8, 4.11, and 4.12 and Chap. 6)*.

It is also important to realise that the end stages of hypoxic-ischaemic brain damage may not become visible until a variable period of time, often several weeks to months after the event, and that the early stages may seem mild or subtle *(Figs. 5.3 and 5.4 and Chap. 6)*. In cases of (suspected) ischaemic injury, even if apparently mild, it is therefore advisable to intensify CUS examinations until normalisation or stabilisation of abnormalities has occurred.

Meningitis and brain infections can have a very rapid, fulminant course and should therefore be intensively monitored by repetitive CUS *(Fig. 5.5)*.

It needs to be emphasised once more that if the timing of CUS is not optimal, the first stages of ischaemic damage may be missed, milder and/or diffuse damage may be overlooked, and complications of haemorrhages or infections may be detected late or not at all. In addition, if CUS examinations are discontinued too early, (the severe end stages of) hypoxic-ischaemic injury may remain undetected.

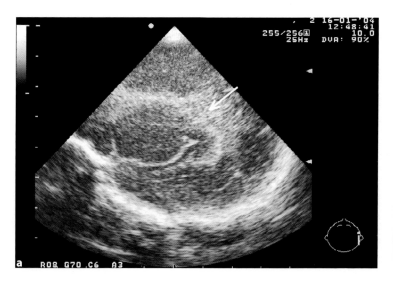

Fig. 5.3a–c Parasagittal ultrasound scan in a preterm infant (GA 31 weeks). **a** Initially show mild, homogenous periventricular flaring (*arrow*) in the parietal region. **b,c** *see next page*

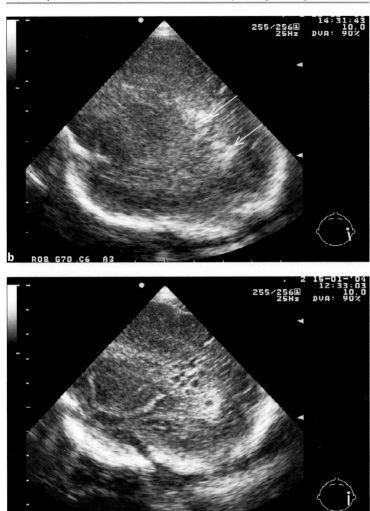

Fig. 5.3 *(continued)* **b** Later evolved into more severe non-homogeneous echodensities (*arrows*) and **c** cystic lesions, which developed only after several weeks

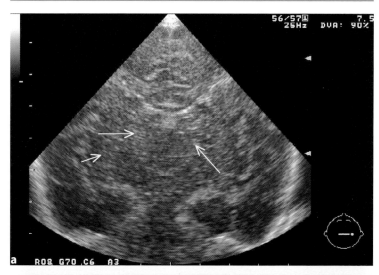

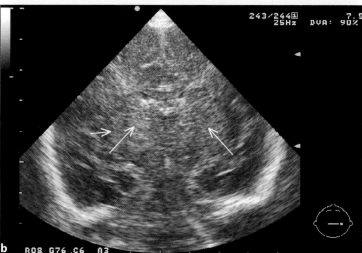

Fig. 5.4a,b Coronal ultrasound scan in a full-term neonate, born asphyxiated. **a** First scan, performed several hours after birth, showing subtle echogenicity in the thalami (*arrows*) and basal ganglia (*short arrows*). **b** On the third day there is more obvious increased echogenicity in the thalamus and basal ganglia, and the brain anatomy is shown in less detail. Compare with normal image as in Fig. 4.1a

Timing of CUS	Background

• Serial examinations until discharge
• Routine screening programme in neonatal units
• Intensify CUS if (suspected) abnormalities
• Term CUS:
  – GA < 32 weeks
  – Birth weight < 1,500 g
  – Suspected parenchymal brain damage
  – Periventricular flaring present at discharge
  – IVH grade 3
  – Complications of IVH
  – Meningitis
  – Brain infections
	• Haemorrhagic lesions:
	  – Early detection (hours)
	  – Occur around birth (< 72 h)
	  – Extension first days after event
	  – Later complications (days/weeks)
	• Ischaemic lesions:
	  – Later detection (hours/days after event)
	  – May develop any time during the neonatal period
	  – Early stages may evolve into late, more severe stages over a long period (weeks/months)
	  – Late detection of end stages
	  – Early stages may seem mild
	  – May be difficult to distinguish from normal phenomena

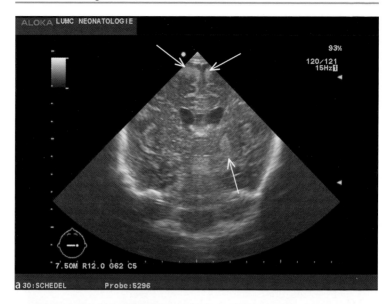

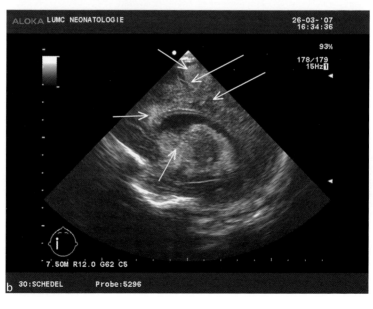

◄ **Fig. 5.5** Ultrasound scan in a 6-week-old full-term infant, 1 week after admittance for group B streptococcal meningitis. This infant initially had normal CUS findings, but eventually developed multi-cystic encephalopathy within a few weeks after the first symptoms of the adequately treated meningitis. **a** Coronal scan at the level of the frontal horns of the lateral ventricles. **b** Parasagittal scan through the left lateral ventricle. CUS shows areas of increased echogenicity (*arrows*), probably presenting infarctions; small areas of ecreased echogenicity (*long arrows*), probably presenting liquefaction; and thickening of the cerebal surface (*short arrows*), probably due to cortical necrosis

Appendix 5.1   Indications for Ultrasonography at Term Corrected Age

- Born prematurely, < 32 weeks and/or birth weight < 1,500 g
- Periventricular leukomalacia ≥ stage 2 according to De Vries et al. *(1992)*
- Periventricular echodensities (flaring) still present at discharge/transfer
- Non-homogeneous periventricular flaring (even if already subsided at discharge/transfer)
- Other lesions of brain parenchyma (such as periventricular haemorrhagic parenchymal infarction, arterial infarction, basal ganglia lesions, brain abcesses, global hypoxic-ischaemic brain damage, etc.)
- P/IVH stage 3 *(Volpe 2001b)* and/or periventricular haemorrhagic infarction and/or post-haemorrhagic ventricular dilatation, needing treatment
- Meningitis or brain infections

References

1.   De Vries LS et al. (1992) The spectrum of leukomalacia using cranial ultrasound. Behav Brain Res 49:1–6
2.   Van Wezel-Meijler G et al. (1998) Magnetic resonance imaging of the brain in premature infants during the neonatal period. Normal phenomena and reflection of mild ultrasound abnormalities. Neuropediatrics 29:89–96
3.   Volpe JJ (2001a) Intracranial hemorrhage: germinal matrix-intraventricular hemorrhage of the premature infant. In: Volpe JJ (ed) Neurology of the newborn. WB Saunders, Philadelphia

Further Reading

1.   Bracci R et al. (2006) The timing of neonatal brain damage. Biol Neonate 90:145–155
2.   Daneman A et al. (2006) Imaging of the brain in full-term neonates: does sonography still play a role? Pediatr Radiol 36:636–646
3.   Davies MW et al. (2000) Reference ranges for the linear dimensions of the intracranial ventricles in preterm neonates. Arch Dis Child Fetal Neonatal Ed 82: F218–F223
4.   De Vries LS, Groenendaal F (2002) Neuroimaging in the preterm infant. Ment Retard Dev Disabil Res Rev 8:273–280
5.   De Vries LS, Levene MI (2001) Cerebral ischemic lesions. In: Levene MI et al. (eds) Fetal and neonatal neurology and neurosurgery. Churchill Livingstone, London
6.   De Vries LS et al. (2004) Ultrasound abnormalities preceding cerebral palsy in high-risk preterm infants. J Pediatr 144:815–820
7.   Huppi PS et al. (1996) Structural and neurobehavioral delay in postnatal brain development of preterm infants. Pediatr Res 39:895–901
8.   Inder TE et al. (2005) Abnormal cerebral structure is present at term in premature infants. Pediatrics 115:286–294
9.   Leijser LM et al. (2006) Using cerebral ultrasound effectively in the newborn infant. Early Hum Dev 82:827–835
10. Levene MI (1981) Measurement of the growth of the lateral ventricles in preterm infants with real-time ultrasound. Arch Dis Child 56:900–904

11. Levene MI, De Vries LS (2001) Neonatal intracranial hemorrhage. In: Levene MI et al. (eds) Fetal and neonatal neurology and neurosurgery. Churchill Livingstone, London

12. Mewes AU et al. (2006) Regional brain development in serial magnetic resonance imaging of low-risk preterm infants. Pediatrics 118:23–33

13. Paneth N et al. (1993) Incidence and timing of germinal matrix/intraventricular hemorrhage in low birth weight infants. Am J Epidemiol 137:1167–1176

14. Paneth N et al. (1994) Brain damage in the preterm infant. Clin Dev Med 131:171–185

15. Pierrat V et al. (2001) Ultrasound diagnosis and neurodevelopmental outcome of localised and extensive cystic periventricular leucomalacia. Arch Dis Child Fetal Neonatal Ed 84:F151–F156

16. Van Wezel-Meijler G et al. (1999a) Unilateral thalamic lesions in premature infants: risk factors and short-term prognosis. Neuropediatrics 30:300–306

17. Van Wezel-Meijler G et al. (1999b) Predictive value of neonatal MRI as compared to ultrasound in premature infants with mild periventricular white matter changes. Neuropediatrics 30:231–238

18. Veyrac C et al. (2006) Brain ultrasonography in the premature infant. Pediatr Radiol 36: 626–635

19. Volpe JJ (1989) Intraventricular hemorrhage in the premature infant – current concepts. II. Ann Neurol 25: 109–116

20. Volpe JJ (2001a) Hypoxic-ischemic encephalopathy: clinical aspects. In: Volpe JJ (ed) Neurology of the newborn. WB Saunders, Philadelphia

21. Volpe JJ (2001c) Intracranial hemorrhage: subdural, primary subarachnoid, intracerebellar, intraventricular (term infant), and miscellaneous. In: Volpe JJ (ed) Neurology of the newborn. WB Saunders, Philadelphia

Classification of Peri- and Intra-ventricular Haemorrhage, Periventricular Leukomalacia, and White Matter Echogenicity

6.1 Scoring Systems

In order to obtain insight into the severity of lesions and for better prognostication, it is recommended that a scoring system be applied for P/IVH, PVL, and periventricular echogenicity. These scoring systems are presented in *Appendices 6.1, 6.2, and 6.3,* respectively.

Appendix 6.1 Classification of Peri- and Intraventricular Haemorrhage

Adapted from Volpe *(1989)*:

- Grade 1: germinal matrix haemorrhage with no or minimal IVH (<10% of ventricular area on parasagittal view) *(Fig. 6.1)*
- Grade 2: IVH (10–50% of the ventricular area on parasagittal view) *(Fig. 6.2)*
- Grade 3: IVH (>50% of the ventricular area on parasagittal view; usually distends to the lateral ventricle) *(Fig. 6.3)*
- Separate notation: concomitant periventricular echodensity (location and extent), referred to as "IPE" (intraparenchymal echodensity), periventricular haemorrhagic parenchymal infarction, or venous infarction *(Fig. 6.4)*
- Separate notation: PHVD *(Fig. 6.5; see also Fig. 6.3c)*

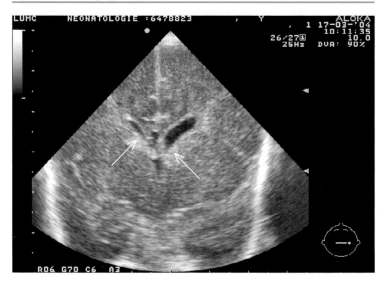

Fig. 6.1 Coronal ultrasound scan in a preterm infant at the level of the frontal horns of the lateral ventricles, showing bilateral germinal matrix haemorrhage (*arrows*; grade 1 P/IVH) and asymmetric ventricular dilatation of the left lateral ventricle

▶ **Fig. 6.2** Grade 2 IVH **a** Coronal ultrasound scan in a preterm baby (GA 26 weeks, scanned at post-conceptional age 29 weeks), level of the bodies of the lateral ventricles, showing bilateral IVH (*arrows*). **b** Parasagittal ultrasound scan through left lateral ventricle (same infant, some days later) showing IVH (*arrows*), beginning PHVD, and increased echogenicity of the ventricular wall (*short arrow*)

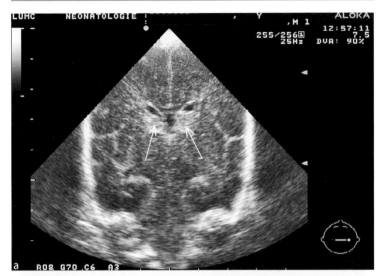

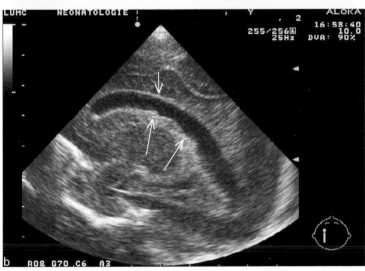

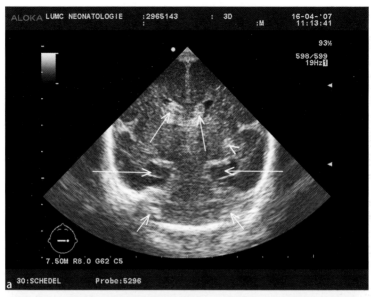

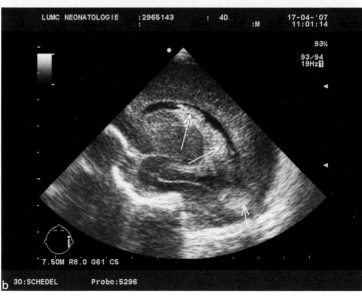

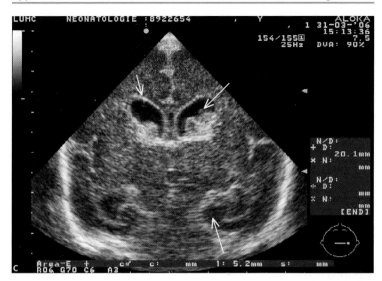

⬅🔼 Fig. 6.3a–c Grade 3 IVH. **a** Coronal ultrasound scan in a preterm neonate (GA 28 weeks, level of the bodies of the lateral ventricles), showing bilateral IVH (*arrows*), distending the frontal and temporal (*long arrows*) horns of the lateral ventricles; also showing echodensities in the cerebellar hemispheres (*short arrows*) and a small echodensity in the area of the left basal ganglia (*arrowhead*), presenting haemorrhages. **b** Parasagittal ultrasound scan through the right lateral ventricle (same infant, 1 day later), showing the large IVH (*arrows*) distending the lateral ventricle and the haemorrhage in the right cerebellar hemisphere (*short arrow*). **c** Coronal ultrasound scan in another preterm infant with grade 3 IVH, showing more obvious dilatation of the frontal and temporal horns of the lateral ventricles (*arrows*), "ballooning" of the frontal horns (grade 3 IVH with PHVD, and increased echogenicity of the ventricular wall (*short arrow*)

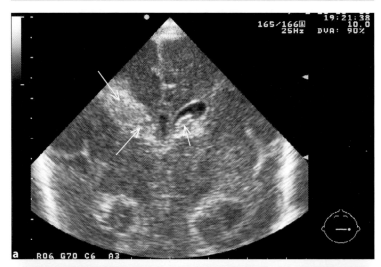

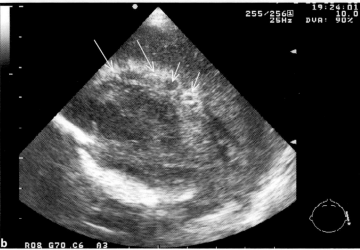

Fig. 6.4a,b Ultrasound scan in a preterm infant with bilateral IVH and right-sided periventricular haemorrhagic infarction (also referred to as venous infarction, or IPE). **a** Coronal scan showing the intraventricular haemorrhages (*short arrows*) and a large echodensity in the right fronto-parietal white matter (*arrow*). **b** Parasagittal scan showing the echodensity (*arrows*) extending from the frontal white matter into the parietal white matter; also beginning to show some echolucency (*short arrows*), presenting cystic degeneration

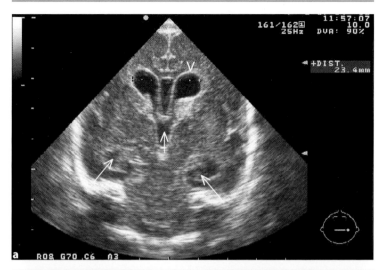

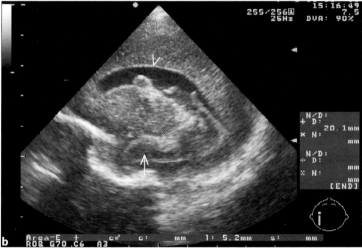

Fig. 6.5a,b Ultrasound scan in a preterm infant with IVH (grade 3) and PVHD. **a** Coronal view showing the haemorrhages, dilated frontal horns, and temporal horns (*arrows*) of the lateral ventricles, dilated third ventricle (*short arrow*), and echogenic ventricular wall (*arrowhead*). **b** Parasagittal view showing IVH, dilated lateral ventricle, and echogenic ventricular wall

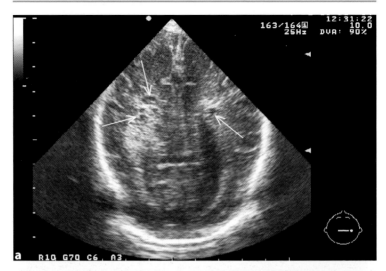

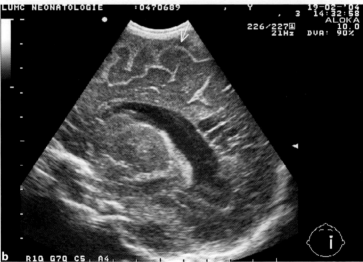

Fig. 6.6a,b Grade 3 PVL. Ultrasound scan in a preterm infant, PCA 34 weeks, born at 29 weeks' gestation, with a complicated course. **a** Coronal view showing cystic lesions surrounded by echodensities in the parietal white matter (*arrows*) (same image as *Fig. 5.2b*). **b** Parasagittal view 1 month later showing extensive cystic lesions in the parietal white matter and also showing dilated lateral ventricle and wide subarachnoidal spaces (*short arrow*), both resulting from tissue loss

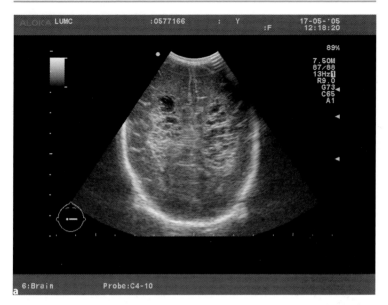

Fig. 6.7a,b Ultrasound scan in a premature infant who gradually, over a period of weeks, developed extensive leukomalacia (grade 4), showing cystic lesions extending into the deep white matter. This baby was one of monochoriotic twins; the pregnancy had been complicated by severe twin-to-twin transfusion syndrome. **a** Coronal view at the level of the parieto-occipital lobes. **b** *see next page*

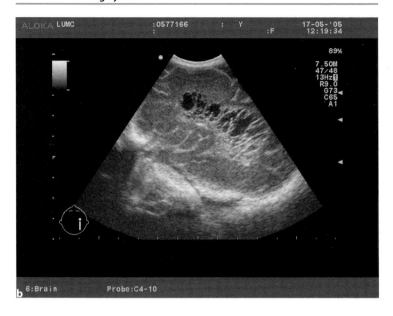

Fig. 6.7a,b *(continued)* **b** Parasagittal view

Appendix 6.2   Classification of Periventricular Leukomalacia

According to de Vries et al. *(1992)*:

- Grade 1: transient periventricular echodensities persisting for ≥ 7 days *(see Figs. 4.5b, 5.1b, 5.2a, 5.3a, and 5.3b)*
- Grade 2: transient periventricular echodensity evolving into small, localised fronto-parietal cysts *(see Fig. 3.6b)*
- Grade 3: periventricular echodensities evolving into extensive periventricular cystic lesions *(Fig. 6.6; see also Figs. 3.2, 5.2b, and 5.3c)*
- Grade 4: densities extending into the deep white matter evolving into extensive cystic lesions *(Fig. 6.7)*

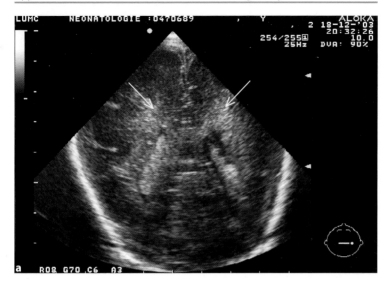

Fig. 6.8a,b Ultrasound scan in a preterm baby with moderately increased echogenicity ("flaring") of the parietal periventricular white matter (grade 1 echogenicity) (*arrows*). **a** Coronal view at the level of the trigone of the lateral ventricles. **b** *see next page*

Appendix 6.3   Classification of Periventricular White Matter Echogenicity

According to van Wezel et al. and adapted according to Sie et al. *(1998, 2000)*:

- Grade 0: normal echogenicity of the periventricular white matter (the echogenicity of the periventricular white matter being less than that of the choroid plexus) *(see Figs. 4.1a, 4.2, 4.3a, 4.5a, and 4.6b)*
- Grade 1: moderately increased echogenicity of the periventricular white matter, the affected region (or smaller areas within the affected region) being almost as bright or as bright as the choroid plexus *(Fig. 6.8; see also Figs. 3.5, 3.10b, 4.5b, 5.1b, and 5.3a)*

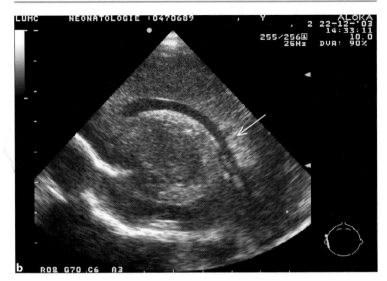

Fig. 6.8a,b *(continued)* **b** Parasagittal view. This infant later developed grade 3 cystic PVL *(same infant as in Fig. 6.6)*

- Grade 2: seriously increased echogenicity, the affected region (or smaller areas within the affected region) being obviously brighter than the choroid plexus *(Fig. 6.9)*
- Separate notation: homogeneous, non-homogeneous *(Fig. 6.10)*

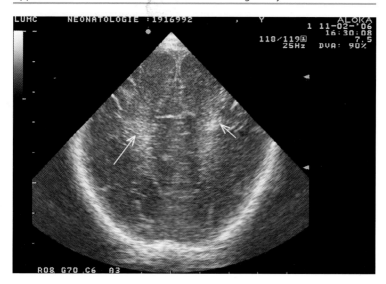

Fig. 6.9 Coronal ultrasound scan in a preterm neonate (GA 31 weeks), showing mainly homogeneously increased echogenicity (grade 1) in the right parietal white matter (*arrow*) and more serious but mainly homogeneously increased echogenicity (echogenicity grade 2) in the left parietal white matter (*short arrow*)

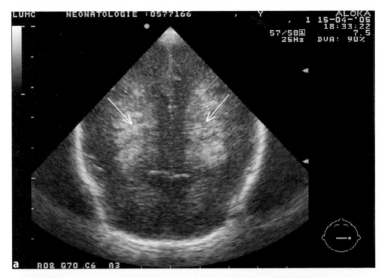

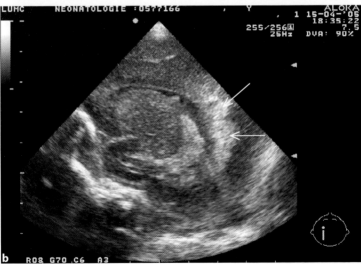

Fig. 6.10a,b Ultrasound scan in a preterm infant, showing diffuse, non-homogeneous, seriously increased echogenicity (grade 2) of the parieto-occipital white matter (*arrows*). This serious periventricular flaring later evolved into extensive cystic PVL (*same infant as in Fig. 6.7, but 1 month earlier*). **a** Coronal view at the level of the parieto-occipital lobes. **b** Parasagittal view through the lateral ventricle

References

1.   Boxma A et al. (2005) Sonographic detection of the optic radiation. Acta Pae-
      diatr 94:1455–1461
2.   De Vries LS et al. (1992) The spectrum of leukomalacia using cranial ultra-
      sound. Behav Brain Res 49:1–6
3.   Sie LT et al. (2000) Early MR features of hypoxic-ischemic brain injury in neo-
      nates with periventricular densities on sonograms. AJNR Am J Neuroradiol
      21:852–861
4.   Van Wezel-Meijler G et al. (1998) Magnetic resonance imaging of the brain in
      premature infants during the neonatal period. Normal phenomena and reflec-
      tion of mild ultrasound abnormalities. Neuropediatrics 29:89–96
5.   Volpe JJ (1989) Intraventricular hemorrhage in the premature infant – current
      concepts. II. Ann Neurol 25:109–116

7.1   Limitations of Cranial Ultrasonography

The advantages of CUS are numerous and widely appreciated *(see Chap. 1)*; however, it is important to acknowledge its limitations:

- Image quality can be affected by small acoustic windows. Although the adaptation of transducer frequency to individual situations and cases and the implementation of additional acoustic windows enhance the possibilities of CUS, some structures and abnormalities remain difficult to visualise.
- Evaluation of superficial structures is difficult; subtle aspects of cortical folding will not be reliably assessed, and extracerebral haemorrhage located at the convexity of the cerebral hemispheres (i.e. subdural, epidural, and subarachnoid haemorrhages) may remain beyond the scope of CUS.
- Cerebellar haemorrhage and infarctions are a well-known complication of very preterm birth and may have important consequences for neurodevelopment. These and other posterior fossa abnormalities are usually detected, especially if additional scanning is performed through the posterior and/or mastoid fontanels, but it is not always possible to define abnormalities precisely.
- Myelination is not visualised.
- Damage to the basal ganglia in term hypoxic-ischaemic encephalopathy and areas of focal infarction are usually detected, but they may not be defined well enough for precise prognostication.
- Diffuse white matter injury, as can occur in very preterm infants, is probably not well detected by CUS.

7.2   Role of MRI

Although MRI cannot replace serial CUS, there are many instances when MRI of the brain is required. MRI depicts brain maturation, including myelination, in much detail. MRI helps to define pathological processes and enables prognostication in many cases. It can help to establish the precise site, origin, and extent of lesions. If abnormalities exist in areas that are difficult to visualise with CUS, MRI may detect lesions that CUS does not. MRI allows detection of diffuse and non-cystic white matter lesions in preterm infants. Modern MRI techniques (diffusion-weighted imaging) allow very early detection of hypoxic-ischaemic brain injury. However, MRI does not enable frequent, serial imaging, and very early imaging within a few hours after birth is hard to realise. In addition, although safe, MRI is much more stressful than CUS for the sick and/or preterm neonate. Some conditions, such as calcifications and lenticulostriate vasculopathy, are better or only depicted by ultrasound.

Thus, in modern neonatology, CUS and MRI are complementary neuro-imaging tools.

7.2.1   Conditions in Which MRI Contributes to Diagnosis and/or Prognosis

- Term hypoxic-ischaemic encephalopathy
- Focal infarction (exact location and extent)
- Periventricular haemorrhagic parenchymal infarction (exact location and extent)
- Diffuse and/or non-cystic white matter damage
- Extracerebral haemorrhage
- Sinus vein thrombosis
- Posterior fossa abnormalities (both congenital and acquired)
- Cortical dysplasia
- Infectious brain disease
- Hypoglycaemia

- Metabolic disease
- Congenital (central nervous system) abnormalities

In *Appendix 7.1*, indications for MRI examinations as applied at our neonatal unit are presented.

7.3   Role of CT

The radiation dose involved in CT scanning is significant, and in most cases CT has little or no additional diagnostic value as compared to high-quality CUS. Therefore, our policy is to apply cerebral CT only under rare conditions, such as suspected calcifications at the brain's convexity, posterior fossa haemorrhage and/or subdural or subarachnoid haemorrhages if intervention is considered and MRI is not readily available, and suspected calcifications at the brain's convexity.

Appendix 7.1   Indications for Neonatal MRI Examinations

- After **perinatal asphyxia:** hypoxic-ischaemic encephalopathy stage 2 or 3 (*Sarnat and Sarnat 1976*) and/or (suspected) CUS abnormalities of the thalami/basal ganglia, cortex, and subcortical white matter. (Optimal timing: days 3–6)
- After **traumatic delivery**
- In newborn infants with **seizures**
- CUS diagnosis of **parenchymal brain injury** (such as cystic PVL, arterial infarction, periventricular haemorrhagic parenchymal infarction, and brain abcesses). Allows exact information on the location and extent of lesions and involvement of the posterior limb of the internal capsule. Best timing in preterm infants: around term corrected age
- In the case of **severe PHVD.** Associated white matter damage? Best timing: around term age.

- Suspected *posterior fossa abnormalities*
- *Miscellaneous:* congenital abnormalities of the central nervous system, congenital malformations, severe hypoglycaemia, congenital infections, infections of the central nervous system, metabolic disorders
- *Extreme prematurity* (< 28 weeks GA) may as such be an indication to perform MRI, preferably around term age. Allows detection of diffuse white matter injury and/or diffuse excessive high-signal intensity in the white matter and evaluation of brain growth and maturation.

References

1.   Sarnat HB, Sarnat MS (1976) Neonatal encephalopathy following fetal distress. A clinical and electroencephalographic study. Arch Neurol 33:696–705

Further Reading

1.   Barkovich AJ (1995) Normal development of the neonatal and infant brain, skull and spine. In: Barkovich AJ (ed) Pediatric neuroimaging. Raven Press, New York
2.   Battin M, Rutherford M (2002) Magnetic resonance of the brain in preterm infants: 24 weeks' gestation to term. In: Rutherford M (ed) MRI of the neonatal brain. WB Saunders, London
3.   Battin MR et al. (1998) Magnetic resonance imaging of the brain in very preterm infants: visualization of the germinal matrix, early myelination, and cortical folding. Pediatrics 101:957–962
4.   Bodensteiner JB, Johnsen SD (2005) Cerebellar injury in the extremely premature infant: newly recognized but relatively common outcome. J Child Neurol 20:139–142
5.   Childs AM et al. (2001) Cerebral maturation in premature infants: quantitative assessment using MR imaging. AJNR Am J Neuroradiol 22:1577–1582
6.   Cowan F et al. (2005) Does cranial ultrasound imaging identify arterial cerebral infarction in term neonates? Arch Dis Child Fetal Neonatal Ed 90:F252–F256
7.   Cowan FM, De Vries LS (2005) The internal capsule in neonatal imaging. Semin Fetal Neonatal Med 10:461–474

8. Debillon T et al. (2003) Limitations of ultrasonography for diagnosing white matter damage in preterm infants. Arch Dis Child Fetal Neonatal Ed 88: F275–F279

9. De Vries LS et al. (1999) Asymmetrical myelination of the posterior limb of the internal capsule in infants with periventricular haemorrhagic infarction: an early predictor of hemiplegia. Neuropediatrics 30:314–319

10. De Vries LS et al. (2005) Prediction of outcome in new-born infants with arterial ischaemic stroke using diffusion-weighted magnetic resonance imaging. Neuropediatrics 36:12–20

11. Limperopoulos C et al. (2005) Cerebellar hemorrhage in the preterm infant: ultrasonographic findings and risk factors. Pediatrics 116:717–724

12. Merrill JD et al. (1998) A new pattern of cerebellar hemorrhages in preterm infants. Pediatrics 102:E62

13. Paneth N (1999) Classifying brain damage in preterm infants. J Pediatr 134:527–529

14. Rutherford M et al. (1996) Hypoxic-ischemic encephalopathy: early and late magnetic resonance imaging findings in relation to outcome. Arch Dis Child 75:F145–F151

15. Rutherford MA et al. (1998) Abnormal magnetic resonance signal in the internal capsule predicts poor neurodevelopmental outcome in infants with hypoxic-ischemic encephalopathy. Pediatrics 102:323–328

16. Rutherford M et al. (2004) Diffusion-weighted magnetic resonance imaging in term perinatal brain injury: a comparison with site of lesion and time from birth. Pediatrics 114: 1004–1014

17. Rutherford M et al. (2006) Magnetic resonance imaging in perinatal brain injury: clinical presentation, lesions and outcome. Pediatr Radiol 36:582–592

18. Rutherford MA et al. (2005) Advanced MR techniques in the term-born neonate with perinatal brain injury. Semin Fetal Neonatal Med 10:445–460

19. Sie LT et al. (1997) MRI assessment of myelination of motor and sensory pathways in the brain of preterm and term-born infants. Neuropediatrics 28:97–105

20. Sie LT et al. (2000) Early MR features of hypoxic-ischemic brain injury in neonates with periventricular densities on sonograms. AJNR Am J Neuroradiol 21:852–861

21. Van der Knaap MS, Valk J (2005) Myelination and retarded myelination. In: van der Knaap MS, Valk J (eds) Magnetic resonance of myelin, myelination, and myelin disorders. Springer, Berlin

22. Van der Knaap MS et al. (1996) Normal gyration and sulcation in preterm and term neonates: appearance on MR images. Radiology 200:389–396

23.   Van Wezel-Meijler G et al. (1998) Magnetic resonance imaging of the brain in premature infants during the neonatal period. Normal phenomena and reflection of mild ultrasound abnormalities. Neuropediatrics 29:89–96

24.   Volpe JJ (2001) Intracranial hemorrhage: subdural, primary subarachnoid, intracerebellar, intraventricular (term infant), and miscellaneous. In: Volpe JJ (ed) Neurology of the newborn. WB Saunders, Philadelphia

25.   Volpe JJ (2003) Cerebral white matter injury of the premature infant – more common than you think. Pediatrics 112:176–180

8   Maturational Changes of the Neonatal Brain

8.1   Maturational Processes

During the late foetal and perinatal period and during early infancy, major maturational processes and growth of the brain take place. Because of this ongoing maturation, the preterm brain in particular is very vulnerable to deviant development and damage. Patterns of perinatal brain injury depend not only on the origin of the injury (i.e. traumatic, hypoxic-ischaemic, inflammatory, haemorrhagic) but also on the PCA of the foetus or infant at the time of the event(s).

Maturational phenomena give very specific CUS features, and CUS images change with ongoing maturation. Those performing neonatal CUS need to be well informed about normal brain maturation, maturational phenomena as depicted on CUS, and (gestational) age-related patterns of perinatal brain injury.

Maturational processes include a major increase in volume, weight, and surface area of the brain; gyration; cell migration; germinal matrix involution; and myelination. These processes can be visualised by modern neuro-imaging techniques, resulting in age-specific features, and will be reviewed in this chapter. Other changes, such as programmed cell death of excess neuroblasts and glioblasts, formation and growth of neurons, and synaptogenesis, are not depicted by neuro-imaging techniques and will not be discussed.

8.2   Gyration

Gyration starts in the second trimester of pregnancy, continues in an ordered, predictable way, and is completed around term age when the brain surface has an almost mature appearance. In extremely preterm infants (GA 24–26 weeks), the brain surface is still very smooth and has a lissencephalic appearance *(Figs 8.1, 8.2)*.

Important regional differences in gyral development exist: Generally, the posterior parts of the brain show the fastest development, and the anterior parts of the brain gyrate much later. Thus, at around 34 weeks of gestation, the frontal cortex can still look very smooth, while the occipital cortex already shows obvious gyration *(Fig. 8.3)*. The process of gyration can be followed by CUS. It is possible to assess the GA of the infant from the ultrasound images.

CUS images of very preterm infants before term age differ substantially from those obtained in infants of around term age, mainly because of the progress in gyration *(see Figs. 8.1, 8.2)*.

While obvious differences in cortical folding between term-equivalent-age preterm and full-term infants as seen on CUS have not been reported, MRI studies have shown that cortical development is not as complex in term-equivalent-age infants born very prematurely as it is in controls born at term.

▷ **Fig. 8.1a,b** CUS scan at the level of the frontal horns of the lateral ventricles. **a** A very preterm infant (GA 26 weeks), showing very smooth cortex (*arrow*) and open insulae (*short arrows*); also showing germinal matrix haemorrhages (*arrow heads*). **b** A term infant showing advanced cortical folding (*arrow*) and closed insulae (*short arrow*)

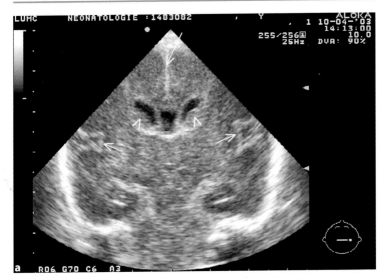

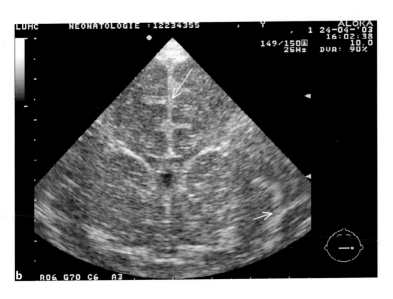

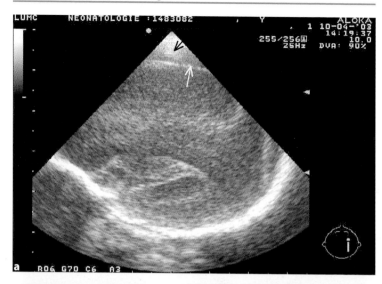

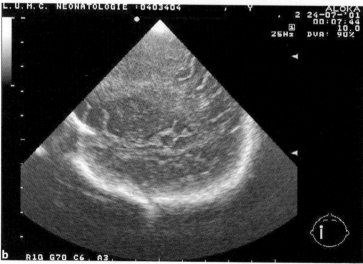

Fig. 8.2a,b Parasagittal ultrasound scan at the level of the insula. **a** The same, very preterm infant as in Fig. 8.1a, showing a smooth cortex (*short arrow*) and absent gyration of the insular cortex. Also shows wide subarachnoid space (*arrow*). **b** A full-term infant, showing advanced development of the insular cortex

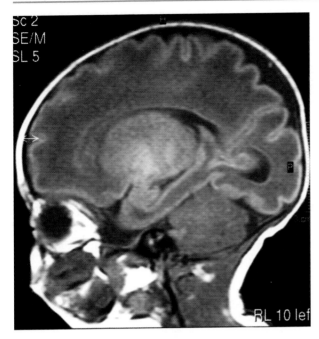

Fig. 8.3 Parasagittal T1-weighted MRI scan in a preterm infant, GA 33 weeks, PCA 34 weeks, showing regional differences in cortical development: The frontal cortex is still almost smooth, while the posterior parietal and occipital cortex show obvious gyration

8.3   Myelination

The posterior brain stem becomes myelinated during the second trimester, but myelination of the anterior brain stem, internal capsule, and cerebral hemispheres does not start until the middle of the third trimester of pregnancy. It then proceeds rapidly during the late foetal period and infancy and continues until early adolescence. Thus, while full-term birth gyration mainly occurs *before* birth, myelination also takes place *after* birth and is very susceptible to perinatal injury.

Like gyration, myelination is a very ordered and predictable process. In general, the central parts of the brain myelinate before the peripheral parts, and the posterior parts before the anterior. Myelination is well depicted by MRI *(Fig. 8.4)* but is not shown on CUS. However, myelination, cell migration, and germinal matrix involution result in white matter changes, which are shown on CUS *(see also Chaps. 4 and 5)*.

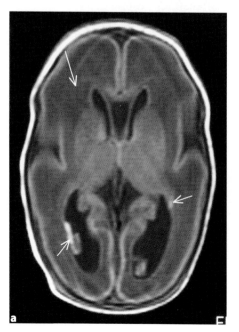

Fig. 8.4a–c Transverse T1-weighted MRI scan at low ventricular level. **a** A preterm infant, GA 28 weeks, scanned at PCA 29 weeks, showing a "watery" brain with low signal intensity of the unmyelinated brain white matter (*arrow*). The basal ganglia have a higher signal intensity than the surrounding unmyelinated white matter. Also shows small germinal matrix haemorrhages (*short arrows*) (movement artefact). **b,c** *see next page*

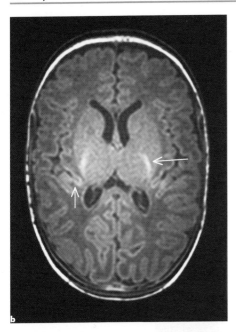

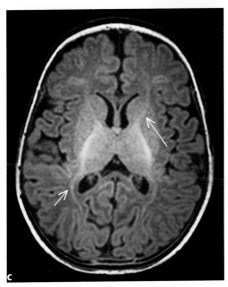

Fig. 8.4a–c *(continued)*
b A full-term neonate, showing a somewhat higher signal intensity of the brain white matter compared with the preterm infant, and obvious myelination (high signal) in the PLIC (*arrow*) and the perirolandic cortex (*short arrow*). Note the advanced cortical development compared with the preterm infant.
c A preterm infant, scanned at 4 months corrected age, now also showing beginning myelination of the anterior limb of the internal capsule (*arrow*) and of the optic radiation (*short arrow*)

8.4   Cell Migration

In the first trimester of pregnancy, neurons migrate towards the immature cortex. Although neuronal cell migration is completed after 20 weeks of gestation, migration of glial cells continues until late gestation. Glial cell migration is visualised on T1- and T2-weighted MR images as regular bands of alternating signal intensity. In normal preterm infants, we may recognise on CUS subtle areas of symmetrical increased echogenicity, mainly in the frontal regions. These areas of increased echogenicity represent glial cell migration and should be distinguished from pathological periventricular flares (see Fig. 5.1).

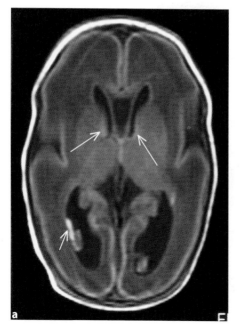

Fig. 8.5a,b Transverse MRI scan at low ventricular level in a preterm infant, PCA 29 weeks (same infant as in Fig. 8.4a), showing germinal matrix, visible as strips in the ventricular wall (*arrows*), having a high signal intensity on the T1-weighted image (**a**) and a low signal on the T2-weighted image (**b**).
see next page

8.5 Germinal Matrix Involution

The germinal matrix is an abundant, highly cellular and vascular "strip" of subependymal tissue. During early gestation it lines the entire wall of the lateral ventricles and third ventricle. It produces neuroblasts and glioblasts and is the origin of migrating neurons (first trimester) and glial cells (second and third trimesters). Regression of the germinal matrix starts from 24–26 weeks of gestation onwards. After 34 weeks, remnants remain in the thalamo-caudate notch and temporal horns of the lateral ventricles. On MR images of preterm infants, the germinal matrix is clearly visible as a high or low signal intensity strip in the ventricular wall on T1- and T2-weighted images, respectively *(Fig. 8.5)*. On CUS, the germinal matrix can be distinguished as small areas of high echogenicity, mostly only visible around the thalamo-caudate notch *(Fig. 8.6)*.

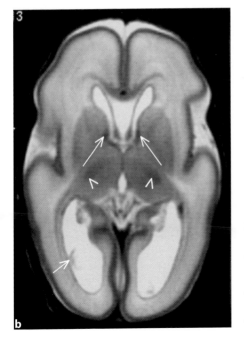

Fig. 8.5 *(continued)* **b** Also shows myelination in the ventral thalamic nuclei (*arrowheads* in **b**) and small germinal matrix haemorrhages (*short arrows*) having high signal intensity on the T1-weighted image (**a**) and lower signal intensity on the T2-weighted image (**b**)

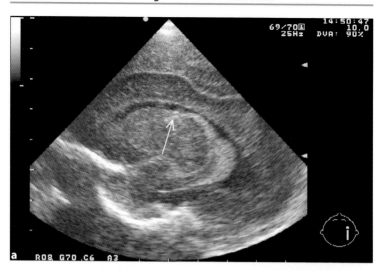

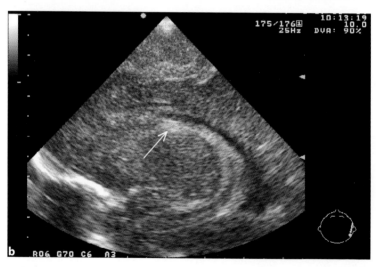

Fig. 8.6a,b Parasagittal ultrasound scan through the right lateral ventricle. **a** A preterm infant, GA 28 weeks, showing remnants of the germinal matrix in the thalamo-caudate notch (*arrow*). This should not be confused with **b** small germinal matrix haemorrhage (*arrow*), often originating at the same location. (preterm infant, GA 29 weeks)

8.6   Deep Grey Matter Changes

On CUS of preterm infants, the thalami and basal ganglia undergo changes. In very preterm infants these deep grey matter structures may show a diffuse, subtly increased echogenicity compared with surrounding tissue *(Fig. 8.7)*. The origin of this phenomenon still needs to be established. It may be the result of changes in myelin and water content within these structures and/or the surrounding tissue, and/or the result of changes in fibre density. This diffuse, subtly increased echogenicity should be distinguished from pathological changes in the deep grey matter resulting from hypoxic-ischaemic injury, typically occuring in (near)-term neonates after perinatal asphyxia *(Fig. 8.8; see also Figs. 2.3 and 4.6a)* and from more localised or unilateral lesions in the thalami and/or basal ganglia, resulting from haemorrhage or infarction in these areas *(see Fig. 4.6c)*.

Therefore, a diffuse, subtle, echogenic "haze" over the basal ganglia and/or thalami can be a normal finding in very preterm neonates, whereas in (near) term neonates, increased echogenicity increase in this same region often presents hypoxic-ischaemic injury, with possible, sometimes serious, consequences for neurodevelopment.

8.7   Changes in Cerebrospinal Fluid Spaces

In the foetus and very preterm infant, the lateral ventricles are often wide and asymmetric (usually the left is larger than the right) with very wide occipital horns *(see Fig. 8.7b)*. Subarachnoid spaces may also be wide *(Fig. 8.9; see also Fig. 8.2a)*. Because of brain growth and loss of fluid in the first few days, the cerebrospinal fluid spaces gradually become smaller. Under some conditions (after extreme prematurity, in infants with congenital cardiac defects, after perinatal asphyxia) the cerebrospinal fluid spaces are sometimes wide, even after term age *(see Fig. 4.9)*. This may be the result of impaired brain growth.

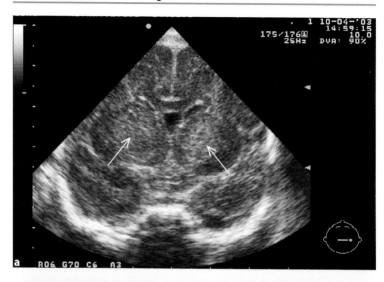

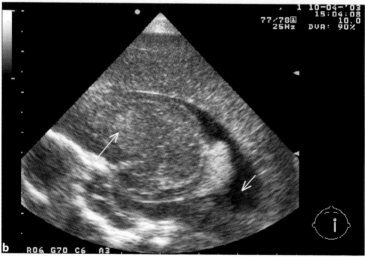

Fig. 8.7a,b Ultrasound scan in a preterm infant, GA 27 weeks, showing diffuse, subtly increased echogenicity in the basal ganglia (*arrows*). **a** Coronal scan at the level of the frontal horns of the lateral ventricles. **b** Parasagittal scan through the lateral ventricle, also showing wide occipital horn of the lateral ventricle (*short arrow*), which is frequently seen in very preterm infants

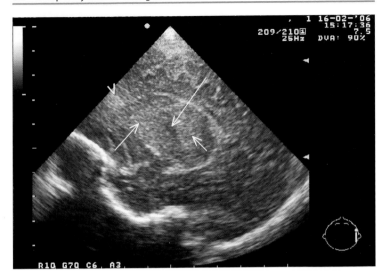

Fig. 8.8 Parasagittal ultrasound scan through the lateral ventricle in a term neonate, born asphyxiated (same infant as in Fig. 4.6a), showing pathological, diffusely increased echogenicity in the basal ganglia (*arrow*) and thalamus (*short arrow*). In between these echogenic structures, the internal capsule stands out as a structure of low echogenicity (*long arrow*). *Arrowhead* shows increased echogenicity in the frontal white matter, an abnormal finding in full-term neonates

Changes of Brain Maturation
• Increase in volume and weight
• Cortical folding
• Myelination
• Cell migration
• Germinal matrix involution
• Deep grey matter changes
• Decrease in cerebrospinal fluid spaces

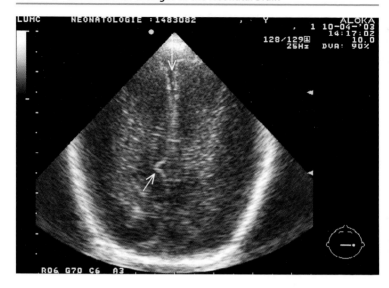

Fig. 8.9 Coronal ultrasound scan in a very preterm infant (same infant as in Figs. 8.1a and 8.2a), at the level of the parieto-occipital lobes, showing wide subarachnoid space (*arrow*). Also shows the onset of calcarine fissure formation (*short arrow*)

Further Reading

1. Barkovich A, Truwit C (1990) Brain damage from perinatal asphyxia: correlation of MR findings with gestational age. AJNR Am J Neuroradiol 11:1087–1096

2. Barkovich AJ, Sargent SK (1995) Profound asphyxia in the premature infant: imaging findings. AJNR Am J Neuroradiol 16:1873–1846

3. Barkovich AJ et al. (1995) Perinatal asphyxia: MR findings in the first 10 days. AJNR Am J Neuroradiol 16:427–438

4. Battin M, Rutherford M (2002) Magnetic resonance of the brain in preterm infants: 24 weeks' gestation to term. In: Rutherford M (ed) MRI of the neonatal brain. WB Saunders, London

5. Battin MR et al. (1998) Magnetic resonance imaging of the brain in very preterm infants: visualization of the germinal matrix, early myelination, and cortical folding. Pediatrics 101:957–962

6.   Boxma A et al. (2005) Sonographic detection of the optic radiation. Acta Paediatr 94:1455–1461

7.   Chi JG et al. (1977) Gyral development of the human brain. Ann Neurol 1:86–93

8.   Childs AM et al. (2001) Cerebral maturation in premature infants: quantitative assessment using MR imaging. AJNR Am J Neuroradiol 22:1577–1582

9.   Counsell SJ et al. (2002) MR imaging assessment of myelination in the very preterm brain. AJNR Am J Neuroradiol 23:872–881

10. Cowan F (2002) Magnetic resonance imaging of the normal infant brain: term to 2 years. In: Rutherford M (ed) MRI of the neonatal brain. WB Saunders, London

11. Davison AN, Dobbing J (1966) Myelination as a vulnerable period in brain development. Br Med Bull 22:40–44

12. De Vries LS et al. (1997) Infarcts in the vascular distribution of the middle cerebral artery in preterm and fullterm infants. Neuropediatrics 28:88–96

13. Horsch S et al. (2005) Ultrasound diagnosis of brain atrophy is related to neurodevelopmental outcome in preterm infants. Acta Paediatr 94:1815–1821

14. Huppi PS et al. (1996) Structural and neurobehavioral delay in postnatal brain development of preterm infants. Pediatr Res 39:895–901

15. Larroche J-C (1987) Le developpement du cerveau foetal humain. Atlas anatomique. INSERM CNRS, Paris

16. Leijser LM et al. (2004) Hyperechogenicity of the thalamus and basal ganglia in very preterm infants: radiological findings and short-term neurological outcome. Neuropediatrics 35:283–289

17. Maalouf EF et al. (1999) Magnetic resonance imaging of the brain in a cohort of extremely preterm infants. J Pediatr 135:351–357

18. Murphy NP et al. (1989) Cranial ultrasound assessment of gestational age in low birthweight infants. Arch Dis Child 64:569–572

19. Naidich TP et al. (1994) The developing cerebral surface. Preliminary report on the patterns of sulcal and gyral maturation – anatomy, ultrasound, and magnetic resonance imaging. Neuroimaging Clin N Am 4:201–240

20. Paneth N (1999) Classifying brain damage in preterm infants. J Pediatr 134:527–529

21. Rados M et al. (2006) In vitro MRI of brain development. Eur J Radiol 57:187–198

22. Sie LT et al. (1997) MRI assessment of myelination of motor and sensory pathways in the brain of preterm and term-born infants. Neuropediatrics 28:97–105

23. Soghier LM et al. (2006) Diffuse basal ganglia or thalamus hyperechogenicity in preterm infants. J Perinatol 26:230–236

24.   Te Pas AB et al. (2005) Preoperative cranial ultrasound findings in infants with major congenital heart disease. Acta Paediatr 94:1597–1603

25.   Van der Knaap MS, Valk J (2005) Myelination and retarded myelination. In: van der Knaap MS, Valk J (eds) Magnetic resonance of myelin, myelination, and myelin disorders. Springer, Berlin

26.   Van der Knaap MS et al. (1996) Normal gyration and sulcation in preterm and term neonates: appearance on MR images. Radiology 200:389–396

27.   Van Wezel-Meijler G et al. (1998) Magnetic resonance imaging of the brain in premature infants during the neonatal period. Normal phenomena and reflection of mild ultrasound abnormalities. Neuropediatrics 29:89–96

28.   Van Wezel-Meijler G et al. (1999) Unilateral thalamic lesions in premature infants: risk factors and short-term prognosis. Neuropediatrics 30:300–306

29.   Veyrac C et al. (2006) Brain ultrasonography in the premature infant. Pediatr Radiol 36:626–635

30.   Volpe JJ (2001) Neuronal proliferation, migration, organization and myelination. In: Volpe JJ (ed) Neurology of the newborn. WB Saunders, Philadelphia

31.   Yakovlev PI, Lecours AR (1967) The myelogenetic cycles of regional maturation of the brain. In: Minkowski A (ed) Regional development of the brain in early life. Blackwell, Oxford

- CUS is an essential diagnostic tool in modern neonatology. It is very suitable for screening, and it depicts normal anatomy, maturational changes, and pathological changes in the brains of preterm and full-term neonates. CUS can reliably be performed only by specially trained individuals and with suitable equipment and technique. CUS plays an important role in assessing neurological prognosis in the infant at risk for deviant development.

- Standard CUS scanning is performed through the anterior fontanel, the whole brain is scanned, and images are recorded in at least six coronal and five sagittal planes with a 7.5-MHz frequency transducer. In individual cases, other frequencies may need to be applied, and scanning through supplemental acoustic windows may be necessary.

- Optimal timing and frequency of serial CUS examinations is essential. It is recommended that screening programmes be applied in neonatal units. Screening schedules should take into account the fact that ischaemic lesions can develop at any time during the neonatal period and may change in appearance over a variable period of time.

- Additional MRI is recommended if parenchymal damage is present or suspected and in very preterm infants, and infants with congenital malformations and miscellaneous disorders. MRI can show the location and extent of lesions more precisely and is better able to depict abnormalities in the posterior fossa. MRI detects subtle or diffuse white matter injury. In addition, MRI gives more detailed information about maturational processes.

- Knowledge of normal anatomy is essential when performing CUS.

- During the late foetal period and in the case of (very) preterm birth, essential maturational processes of the brain take place and can be visualised by modern neuro-imaging techniques. These maturational processes include brain growth, surface development, and enlargement (gyration); white matter changes due to myelination, cell migration, and involution of the germinal matrix; deep grey matter changes; and a decrease in cerebrospinal fluid spaces. Knowledge of brain maturation is essential when performing CUS, and maturational changes need to be distinguished from (mild) pathology.
- Patterns of perinatal brain injury depend, among other things, on the origin of the injury and on the PCA of the infant.

10 **Further Reading**

1. Barkovich AJ (1994) Pediatric neuroimaging, 2nd edn. Raven Press, New York
2. Couture A, Veyrac AL (2001) Transfontanellar Doppler imaging in neonates, 1st edn. Springer, Berlin
3. Govaert P, De Vries LS (1997) An atlas of neonatal brain sonography, 1st edn. MacKeith Press, Cambridge
4. Larroche J-C (1987) Le developpement du cerveau foetal humain. Atlas anatomique. INSERM CNRS, Paris
5. Levene MI et al. (2001) Fetal and neonatal neurology and neurosurgery, 3rd edn. Churchill Livingstone, London
6. Levene MI et al. (1985) Ultrasound of the infant brain, 1st edn. Blackwell, Oxford
7. Paneth N et al. (1994) Brain damage in the preterm infant, 1st edn. MacKeith Press, Cambridge
8. Rutherford MA (2002) MRI of the neonatal brain, 1st edn. WB Saunders, London
9. Van der Knaap MS, Valk J (2005) Magnetic resonance of myelin, myelination, and myelin disorders, 2nd edn. Springer, Berlin
10. Volpe JJ (2001) Neurology of the newborn, 4th edn. WB Saunders, Philadelphia

PART II

ULTRASOUND ANATOMY
OF THE NEONATAL BRAIN

The ultrasound scans shown in this section are normal, considering the gestational age of the infant and the post-conceptional age at scanning, unless stated otherwise.

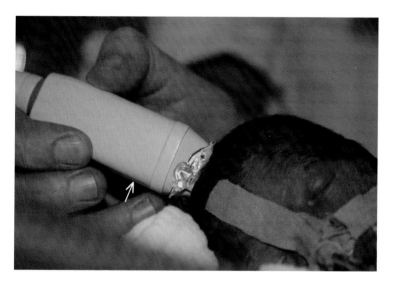

Fig. 1.1 Probe positioning for obtaining coronal planes (*arrow* indicates marker)

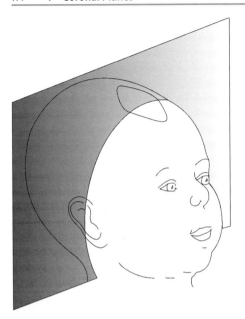

Fig. 1.2 Coronal section

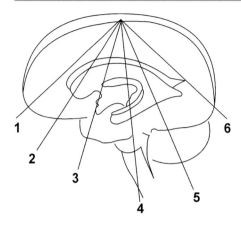

Fig. 1.3 Standard six coronal planes

Legends of Corresponding Numbers in Ultrasound Scans

1. Interhemispheric fissure
2. Frontal lobe
3. Skull
4. Orbit

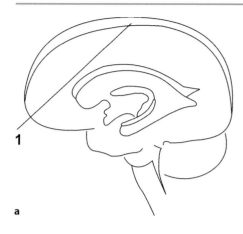

a

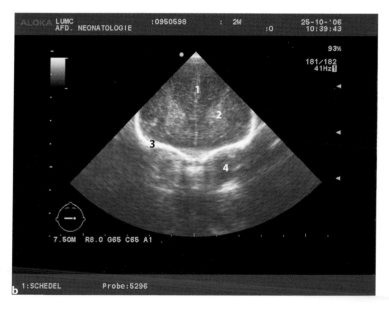

b

Fig. 1.4 a First coronal plane (C1) at the level of the frontal lobes. **b** Ultrasound scan of the first coronal plane (C1) at the level of the frontal lobes (PCA 30 weeks). Scan shows symmetric increased echogenicity of the frontal white matter, a normal finding in preterm infants

Legends of Corresponding Numbers in Ultrasound Scans

1. Interhemispheric fissure
2. Frontal lobe
5. Frontal horn of lateral ventricle
6. Caudate nucleus

7. Basal ganglia
8. Temporal lobe
9. Sylvian fissure

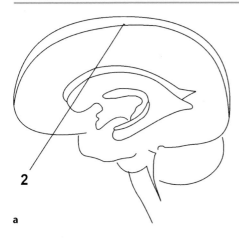

a

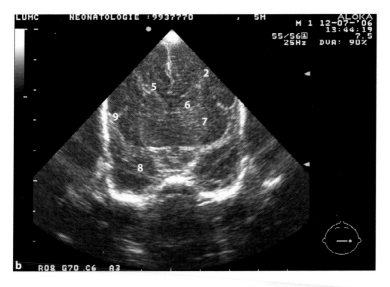

b

Fig. 1.5 a Second coronal plane (C2) at the level of the frontal horns of the lateral ventricles. **b** Ultrasound scan of the second coronal plane (C2) at the level of the frontal horns of the lateral ventricles (GA 27 weeks, PCA at scanning 29 weeks). Ultrasound scan shows subtle, diffuse echogenicity of the basal ganglia, a normal phenomenon at this age

Legends of Corresponding Numbers in Ultrasound Scans

1. Interhemispheric fissure
2. Frontal lobe
5. Frontal horn of lateral ventricle
6. Caudate nucleus
8. Temporal lobe

9. Sylvian fissure
10. Corpus callosum
11. Cavum septum pellucidum
12. Third ventricle
13. Cingulate sulcus

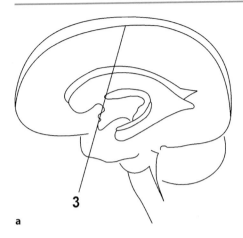

3

a

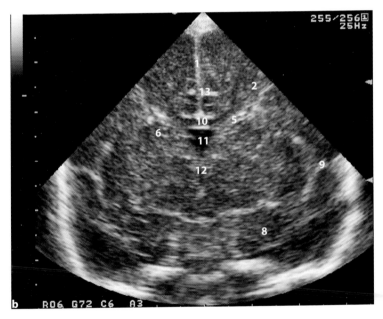

b

Fig. 1.6 a Third coronal plane (C3) at the level of the foramen of Monro and the third ventricle. **b** Ultrasound scan of the third coronal plane (C3) at the level of the foramen of Monro and the third ventricle (PCA 31 weeks); scan shows narrow lateral ventricles, a normal finding if the brain parenchyma has normal echogenicity

Legends of Corresponding Numbers in Ultrasound Scans

1. Interhemispheric fissure
8. Temporal lobe
9. Sylvian fissure
14. Body of lateral ventricle
15. Choroid plexus
    (*: plexus in third ventricle)

16. Thalamus
17. Hippocampal fissure
18. Mesencephalic aqueduct
19. Brain stem
20. Parietal lobe

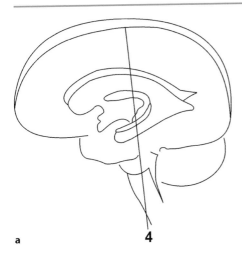

a 4

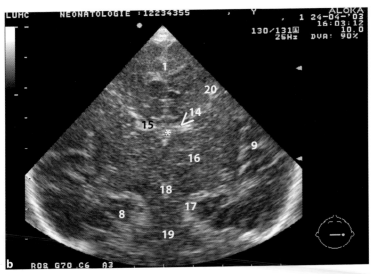

Fig. 1.7 a Fourth coronal plane (C4) at the level of the bodies of the lateral ventricles. **b** Ultrasound scan of the fourth coronal plane (C4) at the level of the bodies of the lateral ventricles (PCA 41 weeks). (Note the advanced cortical folding in this full-term baby)

Legends of Corresponding Numbers in Ultrasound Scans

1. Interhemispheric fissure
8. Temporal lobe
10. Corpus callosum
15. Choroid plexus
    (*: plexus in third ventricle)
20. Parietal lobe

21. Trigone of lateral ventricle
22. Cerebellum
    (a: hemispheres; b: vermis)
23. Tentorium
24. Mesencephalon

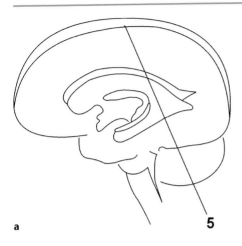

a 5

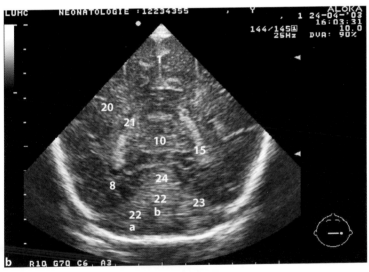

Fig. 1.8 a Fifth coronal plane (C5) at the level of the trigone of the lateral ventricles. **b** Ultrasound scan of the fifth coronal plane (C5) at the level of the trigone of the lateral ventricles (PCA 41 weeks)

Legends of Corresponding Numbers in Ultrasound Scans

1. Interhemispheric fissure
20. Parietal lobe
25. Occipital lobe

26. Parieto-occipital fissure
27. Calcarine fissure

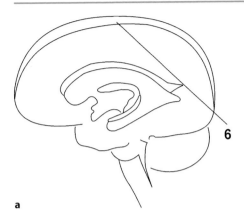

a

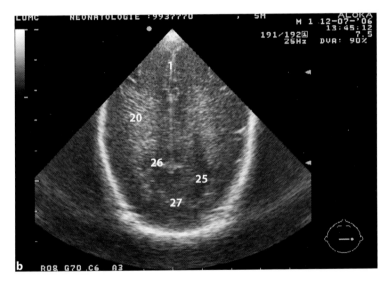

Fig. 1.9 a Sixth coronal plane (C6) through the parieto-occipital lobes. **b** Ultrasound scan of the sixth coronal plane (C6) at the level of the parieto-occipital lobes (PCA 29 weeks)

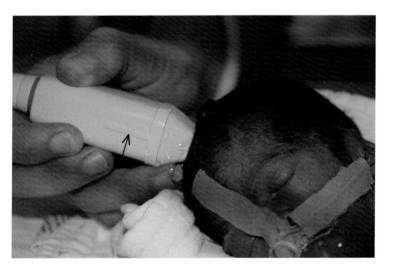

Fig. 2.1 Probe positioning to obtain sagittal planes (*arrow* indicates marker)

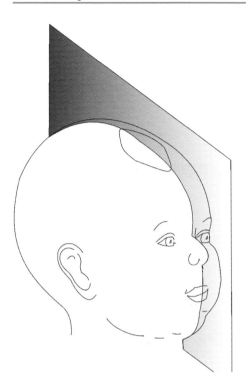

Fig. 2.2 Sagittal section

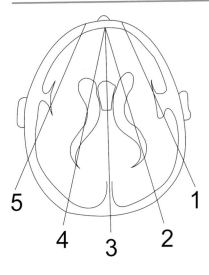

5   1
4 3 2

Fig. 2.3 Standard five sagittal planes

Legends of Corresponding Numbers in Ultrasound Scans

10. Corpus callosum
11. Cavum septum pellucidum
12. Third ventricle
13. Cingulate sulcus
16. Thalamus
22. Cerebellum (b: vermis)
24. Mesencephalon

28. Pons
29. Medulla oblongata
31. Cisterna magna
32. Cisterna quadrigemina
33. Interpeduncular fossa
34. Fornix

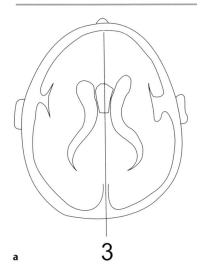

a **3**

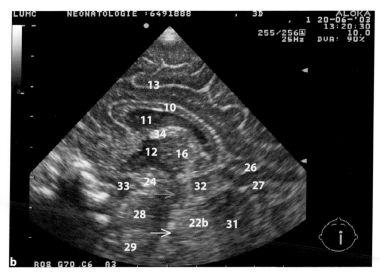

Fig. 2.4 a Midsagittal plane (S3) through the third and fourth ventricles. **b** Ultrasound scan of the midsagittal plane (S3) through the third and fourth ventricle (PCA 40 weeks). *Orange arrow* indicates mesencephalic aqueduct (18). *White arrow* indicates fourth ventricle (30)

Legends of Corresponding Numbers in Ultrasound Scans

2. Frontal lobe
5. Frontal horn of lateral ventricle
6. Caudate nucleus
8. Temporal lobe
14. Body of lateral ventricle
15. Choroid plexus
   (*: plexus in third ventricle)
16. Thalamus

17. Hippocampal fissure
20. Parietal lobe
21. Trigone of lateral ventricle
22. Cerebellum
   (a: hemispheres)
25. Occipital lobe
36. Occipital horn of lateral
   ventricle

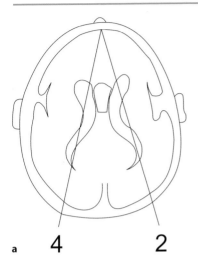

a   4   2

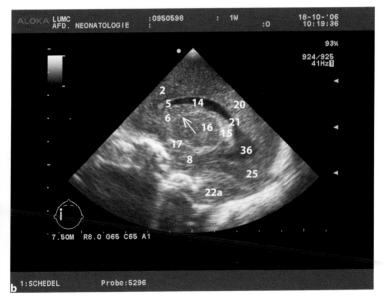

Fig. 2.5 a Second and fourth parasagittal planes (S2, S4) through the right and left lateral ventricles. **b** Ultrasound scan of the fourth parasagittal planes (S4) through the left lateral ventricle (PCA 29 weeks). *Arrow* indicates internal capsule (35)

Legends of Corresponding Numbers in Ultrasound Scans

2. Frontal lobe

8. Temporal lobe

9. Sylvian fissure

20. Parietal lobe

25. Occipital lobe

37. Insula

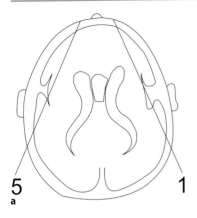

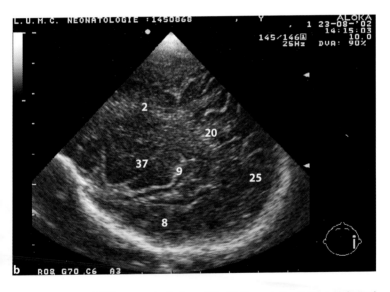

Fig. 2.6 a First and fifth parasagittal planes (S1, S5) through the insulae (right and left). **b** Ultrasound scan of the first parasagittal planes (S1) through the right insula (GA 28 weeks, scanned at PCA 33 weeks)

Posterior Fontanel

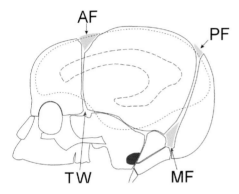

Fig. 3.1 The acoustic windows. *AF* anterior fontanel, *PF* posterior fontanel, *TW* temporal window, *MF* mastoid (or postero-lateral) fontanel

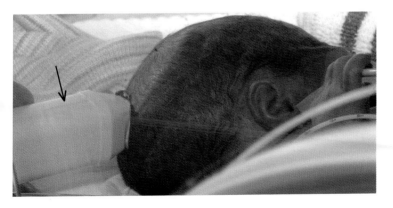

Fig. 3.2 Probe positioning to obtain a coronal view, using the posterior fontanel as an acoustic window (*arrow* indicates marker)

Legends of Corresponding Numbers in Ultrasound Scans

8. Temporal lobe
22. Cerebellum
   (a: hemispheres; b: vermis)
23. Tentorium
25. Occipital lobe
27. Calcarine fissure

29. Medulla oblongata
36. Occipital horn of lateral
   ventricle
38. Falx
39. Straight sinus (sinus rectus)

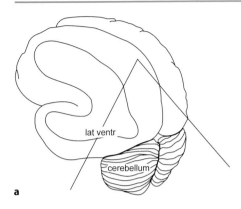

a

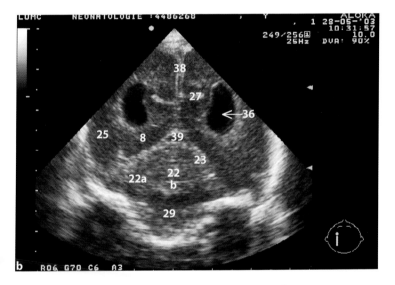

b

Fig. 3.3 a Coronal view, using the posterior fontanel as an acoustic window. **b** Ultrasound scan of the coronal view, using the posterior fontanel as an acoustic window (GA 26 weeks, 5 days, PCA 30 weeks, 2 days). Scan shows wide occipital horns, often seen and a normal finding at this age. Note that the cerebellar vermis is more echogenic than the cerebellar hemispheres

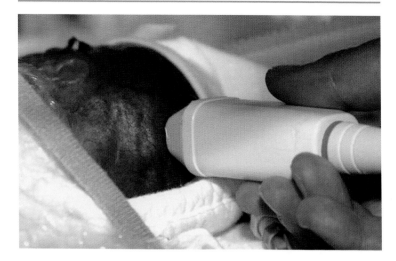

Fig. 3.4 Probe positioning to obtain a sagittal view, using the posterior fontanel as an acoustic window. The marker (not shown here) is on the top of the probe, pointing towards the cranium

Legends of Corresponding Numbers in Ultrasound Scans

8. Temporal lobe
15. Choroid plexus
    (*: plexus in third ventricle)
16. Thalamus
20. Parietal lobe

21. Trigone of lateral ventricle
22. Cerebellum
    (a: hemispheres)
25. Occipital lobe
27. Calcarine fissure

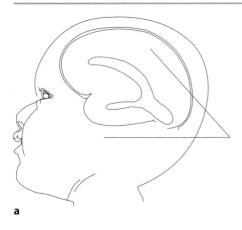

a

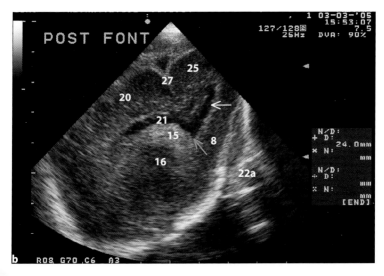

Fig. 3.5 a Parasagittal view, using the posterior fontanel as an acoustic window. **b** Ultrasound scan of parasagittal view through the right lateral ventricle using the posterior fontanel as an acoustic window (PCA 29 weeks, 3 days). *White arrow* indicates occipital horn of lateral ventricle (36). *Orange arrow* indicates temporal horn of lateral ventricle (40)

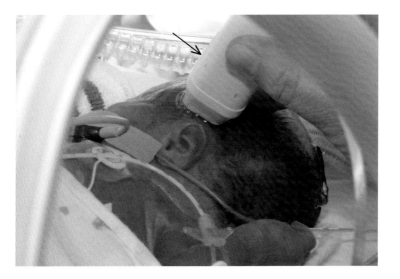

Fig. 4.1 Probe positioning to obtain a transverse view, using the left temporal window (*arrow* indicates marker)

Legends of Corresponding Numbers in Ultrasound Scans

1. Interhemispheric fissure
8. Temporal lobe
12. Third ventricle
22. Cerebellum
   (a: hemispheres; b: vermis)

24. Mesencephalon
33. Interpeduncular fossa
41. Circle of Willis

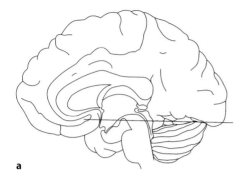

a

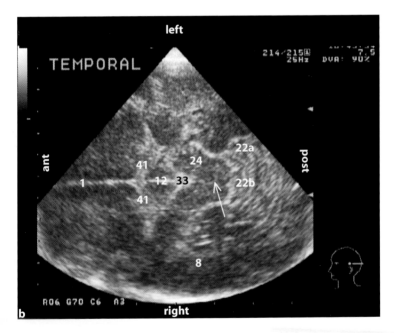

Fig. 4.2 **a** Transverse view using the left temporal window. **b** Ultrasound scan of the transverse view through the upper cerebellum and mesencephalon using the temporal window (PCA 29 weeks, 3 days). *Arrow* indicates mesencephalic aqueduct (18)

Legends of Corresponding Numbers in Ultrasound Scans

8. Temporal lobe
22. Cerebellum
    (a: hemispheres; b: vermis)
25. Occipital lobe

28. Pons
41. Circle of Willis
42. Prepontine cistern

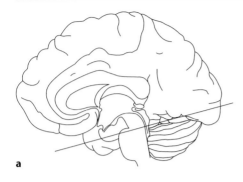

a

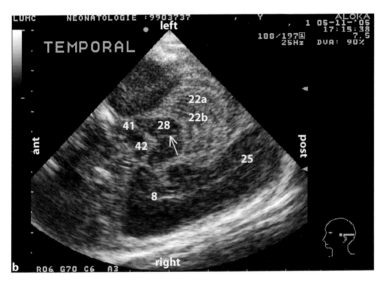

Fig. 4.3 a Lower transverse view using the left temporal window. **b** Ultrasound scan of a lower transverse view through cerebellum and upper pons, using the temporal window (PCA 25 weeks, 2 days). *Arrow* indicates aqueduct of Sylvius (18)

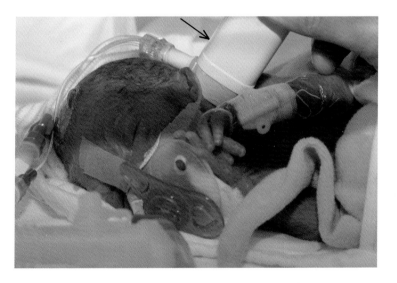

Fig. 5.1 Probe positioning to obtain a coronal view, using the left mastoid fontanel as an acoustic window (*arrow* indicates marker)

Legends of Corresponding Numbers in Ultrasound Scans

22. Cerebellum
    (a: hemispheres; b: vermis)
28. Pons

30. Fourth ventricle
31. Cisterna magna

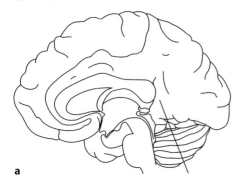

a

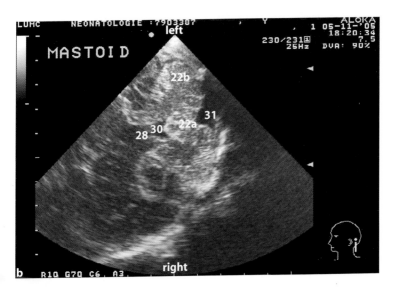

b

Fig. 5.2 **a** Coronal view using the mastoid fontanel as an acoustic window. **b** Ultrasound scan of coronal view through the cerebellum, using the left mastoid fontanel as an acoustic window (PCA 26 weeks). Note that the cerebellar hemisphere further away from the probe shows fewer details than the hemisphere close to the probe (this is normal and should not be confused with pathological changes)

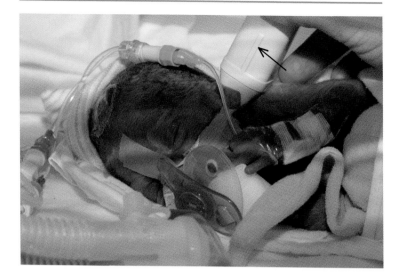

Fig. 5.3 Probe positioning to obtain a transverse view, using the left mastoid fontanel as an acoustic window (*arrow* indicates marker)

Legends of Corresponding Numbers in Ultrasound Scans

8. Temporal lobe
22. Cerebellum
   (a: hemispheres; b: vermis)

25. Occipital lobe
28. Pons

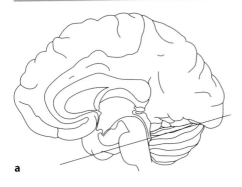

a

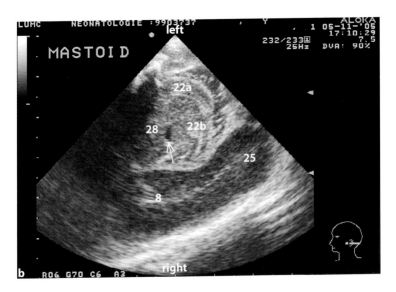

Fig. 5.4 a Transverse view using the mastoid fontanel as an acoustic window. **b** Ultrasound scan of transverse view through cerebellum and pons, using the mastoid fontanel as an acoustic window (PCA 25 weeks). *Arrow* indicates fourth ventricle (30)

Legends of Corresponding Numbers in Ultrasound Scans

1. Interhemispheric fissure
2. Frontal lobe
3. Skull
4. Orbit
5. Frontal horn of lateral ventricle
6. Caudate nucleus
7. Basal ganglia
8. Temporal lobe
9. Sylvian fissure
10. Corpus callosum
11. Cavum septum pellucidum
12. Third ventricle
13. Cingulate sulcus
14. Body of lateral ventricle
15. Choroid plexus
    (*: plexus in third ventricle)
16. Thalamus
17. Hippocampal fissure
18. Aqueduct of Sylvius
19. Brain stem
20. Parietal lobe
21. Trigone of lateral ventricle
22. Cerebellum
    (a: hemispheres; b: vermis)
23. Tentorium
24. Mesencephalon
25. Occipital lobe
26. Parieto-occipital fissure
27. Calcarine fissure
28. Pons
29. Medulla oblongata
30. Fourth ventricle
31. Cisterna magna
32. Cisterna quadrigemina
33. Interpeduncular fossa
34. Fornix
35. Internal capsule
36. Occipital horn of lateral ventricle
37. Insula
38. Falx
39. Straight sinus (sinus rectus)
40. Temporal horn of lateral ventricle
41. Circle of Willis
42. Prepontine cistern

Subject Index

Printing: Krips bv, Meppel, The Netherlands
Binding: Stürtz, Würzburg, Germany